Choosing NSAID Therapy:
An International Reappraisal

Choosing NSAID Therapy:
An International Reappraisal

Guest Editors
F. Dudley Hart
James R. Klinenberg

ADIS Press Limited
USA • United Kingdom • Japan • Hong Kong • Australia • New Zealand

Choosing NSAID Therapy:
An International Reappraisal

National Library of New Zealand
Cataloguing-in-Publication data

Choosing NSAID therapy: an international reappraisal/guest editors, F. Dudley Hart, James R. Klinenberg – Auckland, NZ: ADIS Press, 1985 – 1 v.

ISBN 0-86471-006-2

615.7

1. Anti-inflammatory agents.
I. Hart, F. Dudley (Frank Dudley)
II. Klinenberg, James R.

First printing

ADIS Press
15 Rawene Road, Birkenhead, Auckland 10, New Zealand

Printed in Hong Kong by Dai Nippon Printing Co. Ltd.

Guest Editors

F. Dudley Hart

Honorary Consulting Physician, Chelsea Hospital for Women, Westminster Hospital and Hospital of St John and St Elizabeth, London, England

James R. Klinenberg

Professor and Chairman, Department of Medicine, Cedars-Sinai Medical Center, UCLA School of Medicine, Los Angeles, California, USA

Contributors

Hedley Berry

Consultant Rheumatologist, King's College Hospital, London, England

Peter D. Fowler

Clinical Assistant, Rheumatology Centre, Stoke-on-Trent, Staffordshire, England

F. Dudley Hart

Honorary Consulting Physician, Chelsea Hospital for Women, Westminster Hospital and Hospital of St John and St Elizabeth, London, England

James R. Klinenberg

Professor and Chairman, Department of Medicine, Cedars-Sinai Medical Center, UCLA School of Medicine, Los Angeles, California, USA

Odd Kogstad

Aust-Agder Central Hospital, Arendal, Norway

John M.H. Moll

Consultant Rheumatologist, Sheffield Centre for the Investigation and Treatment of Rheumatic Diseases, Sheffield, England

Alastair G. Mowat

Clinical Lecturer in Rheumatology, University of Oxford and Consultant Rheumatologist, Department of Rheumatology, The Nuffield Orthopaedic Centre, Headington, Oxford, England

Peter A. Simkin

Professor of Medicine, University of Washington, Seattle, Washington, USA

J. Villiaumey

Professor of Medicine, Hospital of Medicine, Hospital Henri Mondor, Paris, France

Frank Wollheim

Professor and Chairman, Department of Rheumatology, University Hospital of Lund, Sweden

Preface

A recent editorial in The Lancet (21 January, 1984), discussing the continuing choice of NSAIDs offered the prescriber, went on to say '. . . the profession must give high priority to continuous education in the process of choosing the most suitable drug and prescribing it in safe and effective quantities.' 'Choosing NSAID Therapy' aims to help not only specialist rheumatologists in their prescribing but also busy general practitioners or hospital internists.

The number of NSAIDs available in the different countries of the world varies greatly, depending largely on the attitudes of regulatory bodies, and it was this fact, as well as a wish to attempt an international consensus that prompted us to invite contributions to this book from rheumatologists of different nationalities. In a series of formal presentations and a final section in the form of a colloquium we have examined the known and postulated properties of NSAIDs. One thing we were in no doubt about: that the availability of a wide choice of NSAIDs contributes to better patient management, for there is great interpatient variability of response and so often Mrs A's wonder-drug is ineffective or not tolerated by Mrs B, and *vice versa*. However, beyond that central fact we have found ourselves on less certain ground, unable, on the available evidence, to say with certainty which features of the NSAIDs confer the benefits and which the disadvantages.

While the search goes on for a better tolerated and more effective agent the doctor needs help in his or her prescribing choice. At present there is no substitute for a careful selection from among those NSAIDs with which the prescriber is most familiar, reserving the newer compounds for patients who fail to respond or who have special problems of intolerance. The NSAIDs remain essential therapy over the whole field of rheumatology and we hope this book will help the reader select the most appropriate agent for any given case.

F. Dudley Hart
James R. Klinenberg

List of Contents

1. Treatment of Rheumatic Disease
The Doctor's Dilemma

James R. Klinenberg

Department of Medicine, Cedars-Sinai Medical Center, UCLA School of Medicine, Los Angeles, California

Factors to Consider

The drug treatment of rheumatic diseases has always been – and continues to be – 'the doctor's dilemma'. There are many factors which make drug treatment of rheumatic diseases so complicated, some of which are:

1) The rheumatic diseases represent over 150 distinct and diverse conditions with very different etiologies, pathogeneses, expressions of symptoms and, therefore, rationales for therapy. In many instances the answers are still not entirely known: for example, how important is it to suppress inflammation in a condition like osteoarthritis which is primarily degenerative? Is pain an important protective device in the rheumatic diseases, and will relief of pain alone prevent patients from recognizing the severity of their joint problem thus causing further destruction by overuse (similar to the Charcot joint)? Under what circumstances do various types of agent actually influence the natural history of the disease, i.e. are the drugs serving purely as symptomatic relief or are they really providing substantive alteration in the disease process?

2) The natural history of many of the rheumatic diseases includes frequent exacerbations and remissions. Thus, it is very difficult to assess the influence of drugs, particularly if they are given over short periods of time (chapter 2), because one must always dissociate the natural variations of the disease from the effect of the drug itself. This occurrence is so common in many of the rheumatic diseases (e.g. rheumatoid arthritis, systemic lupus) that it necessitates carefully controlled studies in order to evaluate the efficacy of any particular drug.

3) Drug use in the management of rheumatic diseases is frequently associated with toxicity. This can vary from the common side effects (chapter 4) of nausea and headache associated with the non-steroidal, anti-inflammatory drugs (NSAIDs) to the serious side effects (chapter 3) of bone marrow suppression, overwhelming infection, and even death associated with the more potent cytotoxic or immunosuppressive agents. This immediately raises the therapeutic dilemma of the substitution of one set of symptoms for another and whether it is a worthwhile exchange. In addition, it raises the important philosophical issue of whether potentially lethal drugs should be used in patients who have debilitating but not life-threatening illnesses.

These are just a few of the issues which make the drug management of rheumatic diseases difficult and at times controversial. In this chapter some of the options will be presented but it should be remembered that in every instance the final decision regarding treatment will be one taken by the physician in conjunction with the patient.

Indications for Drug Treatment

From among the many rheumatic diseases several of the most common have been selected for discussion. They represent well over 90% of rheumatic conditions likely to be seen by a practitioner in the office or in the hospital. This brief review is intended only to put into perspective the spectrum of illnesses treated medically as well as the rationale for therapy.

Osteoarthritis

Pathogenesis

Osteoarthritis is primarily a degenerative disorder. Although the exact etiology is still unknown it would appear that the pathogenesis includes some biochemical, endocrinologic, and/or aging phenomena which cause alteration of the articular cartilage. As a result of these changes the cartilage becomes fragmented and gradually eroded. In an abortive attempt to regenerate cartilage there is new bone formation resulting in the spurs and hypertrophic changes so often seen as part of the basic pathology in osteoarthritis. Thus, the major mechanisms for symptom production in osteoarthritis include loss of articular cartilage, with roughened and often denuded surfaces rubbing on each other causing crepitation, loss of motion, pain, and hypertrophic changes. These can result in spurs, Heberden's nodes, Bouchard's nodes, etc., which cause pressure phenomena and secondary neuropathic changes or muscle spasms.

Symptoms

The symptoms associated with osteoarthritis of the hip or knee are frequently mechanical and related to the loss of cartilage and the rubbing of bone on bone. Symptoms associated with osteoarthritis of the spine may arise from the hypertrophic changes causing occlusion of the neural foramina and subsequent nerve root compression resulting in neuropathic symptoms.

Management

Since there are no drugs able to induce appropriate new cartilage formation, nor any capable of dissolving hypertrophic spurs, there is no definitive drug therapy for the correction of osteoarthritis. Management is, therefore, symptomatic. The definitive treatment of osteoarthritis is often surgical with appropriate use of either osteotomy or total joint replacement.

Anti-inflammatory Agents

Although osteoarthritis is not primarily an inflammatory disorder, there is now good evidence that secondary inflammation does occur in association with this disease. In part, this inflammation occurs because small pieces of cartilage from the deteriorating joint are cast into the joint space where they set up an inflammatory reaction in the synovium (similar to crystal-induced arthritis). This helps explain why patients with osteoarthritis occasionally have acute painful, warm, red swelling of the joint when the synovial fluid may show inflammatory changes.

There is, therefore, a rationale for the use of anti-inflammatory agents in osteoarthritis for the relief of this secondary inflammation as well as for their analgesic effect. This is still only symptomatic management, however, since it does not alter the basic disease process.

The use of intra-articular injections of corticosteroids may bring about temporary resolution of secondary inflammation and result in symptomatic improvement in the patient. However, studies in animals have shown that long-acting corticosteroids introduced into the joint space, especially if part of the material becomes embedded in cartilage, seem to cause even more rapid dissolution of the cartilage. Thus, intra-articular injections into small or large joints, especially if carried out repeatedly, may have harmful consequences.

Non-steroidal anti-inflammatory drugs are the mainstay of treatment for the inflammatory component of osteoarthritis – corticosteroids having far too many side effects to be justified in this setting.

Analgesic Agents

Most NSAIDs have both anti-inflammatory and analgesic properties and it has been suggested that the major benefit in osteoarthritis may be the analgesic effect. Agents with more analgesic than anti-inflammatory activity may bring about more relief in some patients with osteoarthritis.

Again, it should be emphasized that there is no evidence that these agents influence the long term course of osteoarthritis in a positive way. Some workers have even suggested that the symptomatic relief of pain in osteoarthritis is harmful, since it causes the patient to use the joints more frequently and, therefore, may speed their destruction. There is, however, relatively little evidence in support of this concept.

Crystal-induced Arthritis

The major disease caused by crystal deposition is gout. Gout has been recognized and written about for centuries and since the days of Hippocrates it has been known that colchicine, an extract of the autumn crocus, was effective in the symptomatic management of this time-honored condition.

Pathogenesis of Gout

Primarily a disease of men, gout is characterized by a very sudden onset of an acute and intense inflammation, often affecting the great toe (podagra) but although it usually affects a single joint it occasionally involves a few, and rarely, multiple joints. It is often precipitated by some stressful situation.

For the past 200 years, it has been known that gout is associated with hyperuricemia. Many of the factors involved in the deposition of urate crystals in patients with gout are not fully understood, although the concentration of urate, the pH, the temperature, the ionic strength and the nature of the proteins at the site of precipitation are known to be of importance. There is general agreement that during the acute attack of gout, microcrystals of sodium urate are deposited from hyperuricemic body fluids into various tissues, including the synovium and cartilage.

The acute attack of gout involves at least five sequential phases (fig. 1.1):

1) *Precipitation of sodium urate crystals.* Urate crystals are negatively charged and are readily coated by a variety of proteins. Coating with IgG has been shown to stimulate the neutrophil response to crystal formation.

2) *Polymorphonuclear leukocyte response.* Formation of crystals results in the production of a chemotactic factor which causes a polymorphonuclear leukocyte response. There is, however, no direct reaction between the crystal and the leukocyte until the crystal has been phagocytosed in the next phase.

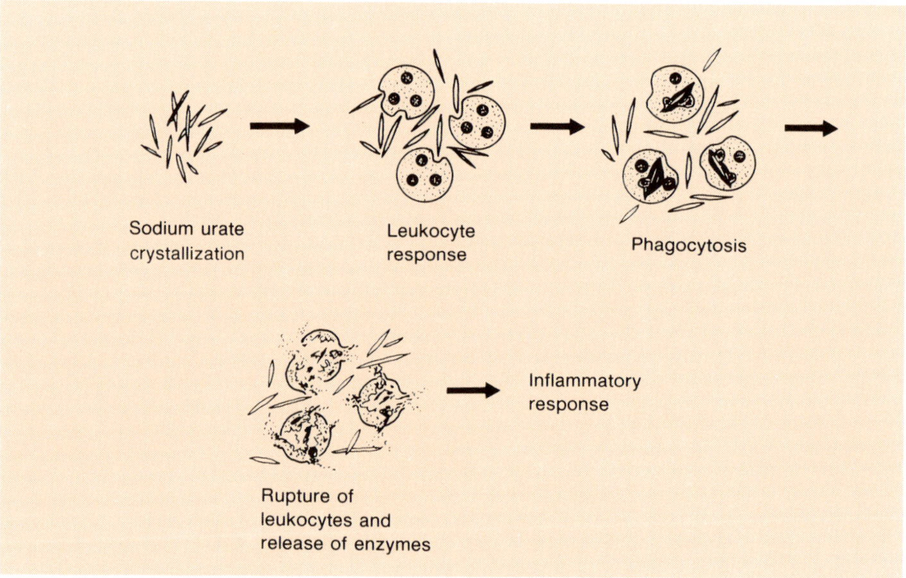

Fig. 1.1. The sequence of events involved in the development of an acute attack of gout in response to the formation of sodium urate crystals.

3) *Phagocytosis.* The crystal is phagocytosed by the leukocyte (fig. 1.2a) with the development of a phagolysosome. Ultimately, the vacuolar membrane surrounding the crystal merges with that of the leukocytic lysosome (fig. 1.2b).

4) *Disruption of lysosome.* After any protein coating of the crystal has been digested, formation of chemical bonds between the surface of the crystal and the lysosomal membrane leads to rupture of the lysosomal membrane and release of enzymes and superoxide radicals into the cytoplasm (fig. 1.2c).

5) *Disruption of the cell.* When disruption of the cell occurs, lysosomal enzymes are released into the synovial fluid, resulting in an increased intensity of the inflammatory response and increased tissue irritation (fig. 1.1 and fig. 1.2d).

These enzymes are also capable of activating a number of inflammatory mediators including the vasoactive polypeptide kinin system, the prostaglandin system and complement, thereby leading to the release of chemotactic factors and an enhanced polymorphonuclear leukocyte response. In addition, these local changes result in a fall in tissue pH and decreased solubility of uric acid crystals which causes further local deposition of urate crystals. Thus, an inflammatory cascade induced by crystal deposition ensues.

Treatment of Gout

The rationale for therapy of crystal-induced arthritis is the suppression of inflammation induced by the crystals, thus stopping the inflammatory cascade. Since colchicine specifically interferes with this reaction, it very effectively relieves the acute symptoms associated with gout. However, as colchicine has considerable toxicity and is not well tolerated by many patients, phenylbutazone, the first of the NSAIDs (after salicylates), became one of the prime agents for the management of gout. Subsequently, each of the new NSAIDs has been found to be very effective in the management of the acute gouty attack. It is usually necessary to begin treatment early with the maximum recommended dosage of the drug (see also chapter 6) in order to achieve rapid cessation of the attack.

The complications of gout, namely, deposition of uric acid in soft tissues (tophi) and in the interstitial areas of the kidney, are consequences of the limited solubility of uric acid in biological fluids, and may be prevented by drug treatment. The uricosuric agents probenecid, benzbromarone and sulfinpyrazone increase urinary excretion of uric acid, and the xanthine oxidase inhibitor allopurinol, blocks uric acid production.

In some elderly patients, especially those with evidence of degenerative joint disease, there is deposition of calcium pyrophosphate crystals and these also are capable of setting up an inflammatory reaction. Crystal-induced arthritis associated with calcium pyrophosphate deposition disease is called 'pseudogout' and is manifest by acute inflammation usually of a large weight-bearing joint in a patient who does not have hyperuricemia. On x-ray the joint shows evidence of calcification of cartilage (chrondrocalcinosis). This crystal-induced arthritis also responds to NSAIDs.

Rheumatoid Arthritis

Pathogenesis

Rheumatoid arthritis is manifest by acute and chronic inflammation of the synovium. It is one of the more common rheumatic diseases, especially in women. For unknown reasons, possibly related either to infection, immunologic mechanisms, or both, patients with rheumatoid arthritis develop inflammation of the synovial membrane which, instead of being a thin glistening membrane only one cell thick, is invaded by both mononuclear cells and polymorphonuclear leukocytes becoming an angry mass of inflammatory tissue which is capable of eroding its way into articular cartilage resulting in destructive changes in the joint (pannus formation). Thus, the articular changes in rheumatoid arthritis are secondary to this active, invasive synovitis. This inflamed synovium is responsible for the symptoms, including pain, warmth, swelling and tenderness of the joint. It is also responsible for an elaboration of excessive amounts of synovial fluid and is capable of causing secondary changes such as tendon rupture or nerve entrapment. Other associated changes take place, including elevation of the sedimentation rate and production of the antiglobulin known as rheumatoid factor.

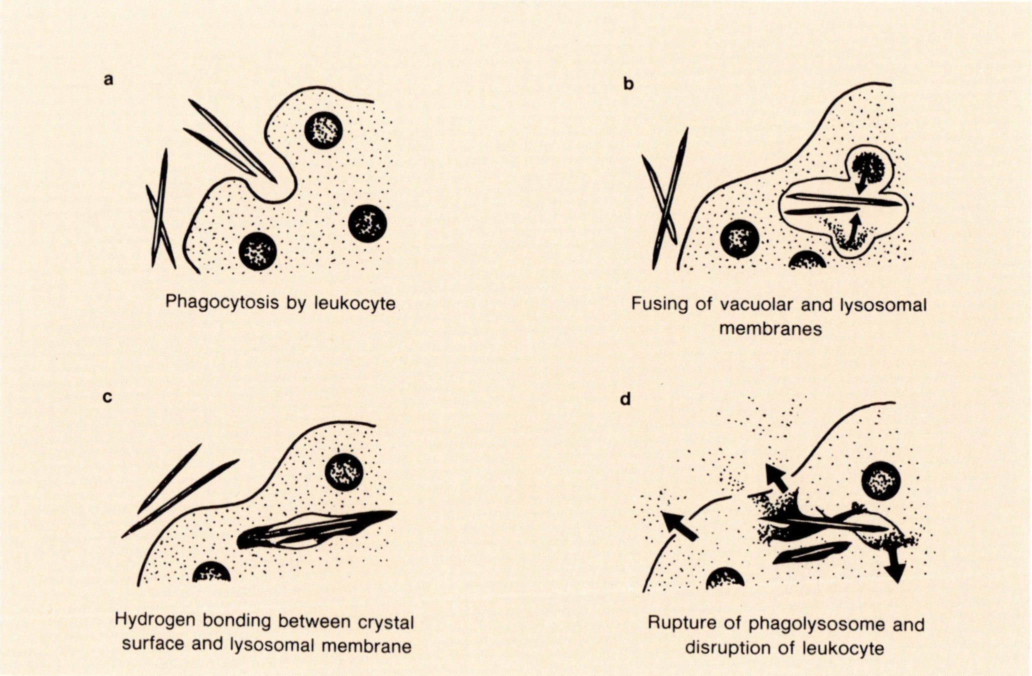

Fig. 1.2. The interaction between leukocytes and urate crystals.

Management

In rheumatoid arthritis the basic pathophysiology is associated with acute inflammation and obviously therapy must be related to suppression of that inflammation. During the past several centuries the search has continued for appropriate anti-inflammatory drugs for the treatment of rheumatoid arthritis.

Corticosteroids

The discovery of corticosteroids in the 1940s began a new era in anti-inflammatory therapy. Hench and his colleagues used steroids in the management of rheumatoid arthritis and the results were so dramatic that they received the Nobel Prize for their work. However, it subsequently became apparent that corticosteroids had very significant toxicity, especially when used in a chronic disease such as rheumatoid arthritis and, in addition, there was little evidence that corticosteroids actually halted the natural progression of the disease.

NSAIDs

The use of salicylates in rheumatoid arthritis had again been known for several decades and aspirin was – and continues to be – the first line of defense in the management of rheumatoid arthritis. When salicylates are given in large doses to achieve blood levels of 20 to 25 μg/dl (just below the level which causes tinnitus), there is considerable evidence of suppression of inflammation and improvement in the patient's symptoms. However, because such large doses of aspirin are often poorly tolerated, the advent of the other NSAIDs has proved a real boon in the treatment of these patients.

All of the NSAIDs have been shown to be effective in certain patients and selection of one rather than another is a matter of balancing efficacy versus toxicity in given patients. For that reason it is important that there are a large number of NSAIDs available to enable the physician to choose the one which the patient tolerates best and which is the least toxic. Unfortunately, at present there seems to be no way to predict which drug patients are most likely to respond to, or with which group of drugs they are more likely to have side effects (see chapter 7). There seems to be very little, if any, evidence that any of the NSAIDs are actually capable of altering the natural history of the disease by reducing the number of erosions which occur in the joints over long periods of time.

Slow-acting Antirheumatic Drugs (SAARDs)

Approximately 20 to 25% of patients with rheumatoid arthritis may have a spontaneous remission within a period of one year after onset of the disease. During this time NSAID treatment is useful. However, if the patient does not have a spontaneous remission and continues to have evidence of active, progressive and destructive disease beyond one year, use of the slow-acting antirheumatic drugs (SAARDs) must be considered.

Drugs in this category include: the antimalarials (especially hydroxychloroquine), gold salts and penicillamine.

Cytotoxic Therapy

If the patient either fails to respond to SAARDs, or develops severe side effects, it may then be necessary to consider the use of cytotoxic or immunosuppressive therapy. There have been some very favorable reports of the use of cyclophosphamide in the treatment of rheumatoid arthritis, again raising the philosophic issue of the potential toxicity of the drug relative to the comparatively benign, although crippling nature of rheumatoid arthritis. Although certain guidelines have been established for the use of cytotoxic therapy in rheumatic diseases, one must also consider the quality of life, remembering that there are significant numbers of patients with rheumatoid arthritis of such severity that use of this type of drug is warranted if all else fails.

Numerous controlled studies have shown good results with azathioprine as well as with cyclophosphamide, and more recently methotrexate and chlorambucil have been used. It has been suggested that combination therapy, such as hydroxychloroquine, gold and azathioprine, might enable smaller doses of the drugs to be used and result in greater efficacy with less toxicity. Other forms of therapy are now under investigation, including plasmapheresis and lymphocyte depletion, either by lymphopheresis or total lymphoid irradiation.

Collagen Vascular Disease

Systemic lupus, dermatomyositis, scleroderma and polyarteritis are systemic diseases in which there may be a significant component of inflammatory arthritis. Each of these conditions can present with a migratory polyarthritis which during the first 3 to 4 months of illness is indistinguishable from the inflammatory arthritis seen in rheumatoid arthritis.

Management

Since many of these illnesses are potentially life-threatening, potent agents such as high-dose corticosteroids or immunosuppressive therapy may be required. However, in many patients arthritis is the major component of their disease and they often benefit from salicylate or NSAID therapy. If, for example, a patient has systemic lupus with only joint manifestations, or with joint manifestations and pericarditis, the use of salicylates or NSAIDs may be all that is necessary for the suppression of the symptomatic portion of the disease. However, if there is renal involvement corticosteroid or immunosuppressive therapy is indicated. The patient with systemic lupus who has only polymorphous light eruption and arthritis may well benefit from therapy with hydroxychloroquine and symptomatic management with NSAIDs.

The Spondyloarthropathies

It has been known for many years that a number of patients have inflammatory arthritis that has some vague resemblance to rheumatoid arthritis, but is obviously different. These conditions (known as the rheumatoid variants) primarily affect men, usually during their late teens or early twenties and thirties, and are associated with an asymmetrical inflammatory arthritis, frequently of the lower extremities but also involving the sacroiliac joints and the axial skeleton. These patients tend to have a very acute onset of disease and are usually seronegative. The spondyloarthropathies include ankylosing spondylitis, Reiter's syndrome, the arthritis associated with psoriasis, and that associated with inflammatory bowel disease.

Long after these conditions had been defined clinically as the spondyloarthropathies (because of the involvement of peripheral joints and spine), it was found that many of these patients had a common human leukocyte antigen, HLA-B27. Thus, approximately 90% of patients with ankylosing spondylitis and Reiter's syndrome are HLA-B27 positive, and this group of diseases is now sometimes referred to as the HLA-B27 arthritides.

Response to NSAIDs

The other characteristic feature of this group of inflammatory arthritides is the dramatic response to NSAIDs. This makes accurate diagnosis important, especially when the back is involved – often the lumbar and thoracic but also the cervical areas. Controlled studies have shown that patients with ankylosing spondylitis responded more effectively to phenylbutazone than to large doses of salicylate.

Non-articular Rheumatism

A large number of patients present with musculoskeletal pain syndromes – both acute and chronic – which are not associated with arthritis *per se* but rather with inflammation of the bursa or the tendon. Bursitis and tendinitis are common causes of musculoskeletal pain and are frequently confused with true arthritis. Acute bursitis or tendinitis is associated with inflammation and NSAIDs are very effective. With very local disease it is sometimes effective to inject the bursa or tendon sheath with corticosteroids but suppression with NSAIDs brings about good symptomatic relief of recurrent or chronic disease. Another large group of patients has a nonspecific musculoskeletal pain syndrome, frequently referred to as fibromyositis or fibromyalgia, with many associated tender points or trigger points. These patients also benefit symptomatically from the use of NSAIDs together with appropriate patient education and the prescription of an effective exercise program.

Mode of Action and Classification of the NSAIDs

Strictly speaking, salicylates were the first NSAIDs, although of course the term non-steroidal anti-inflammatory drug was coined only when the limitations of corticosteroids were recognized and the search for safer drugs embarked on. Phenylbutazone was the first of the new compounds, introduced in the 1950s, followed by indomethacin then, over more recent years, many others (table 1.1).

Mode of Action

NSAIDs probably have many actions, as well as being analgesic and anti-inflammatory. Evidence now suggests that the major mechanism by which the NSAIDs exert their anti-inflammatory effect is by the inhibition of prostaglandin synthesis. Prostaglandins, particularly of the E series, are capable of producing inflammation, and inhibition of this prostaglandin-induced inflammation is probably the major function of the NSAIDs.

Arachidonic acid is the precursor substrate for both cyclo-oxygenase (prostaglandin synthetase) and the lipoxygenase enzymes (fig.1.3). Cyclo-oxygenase then catalzyes the conversion of arachidonic acid to prostaglandins F, D and E, as well as prostacyclin and the thromboxanes. Lipoxygenase

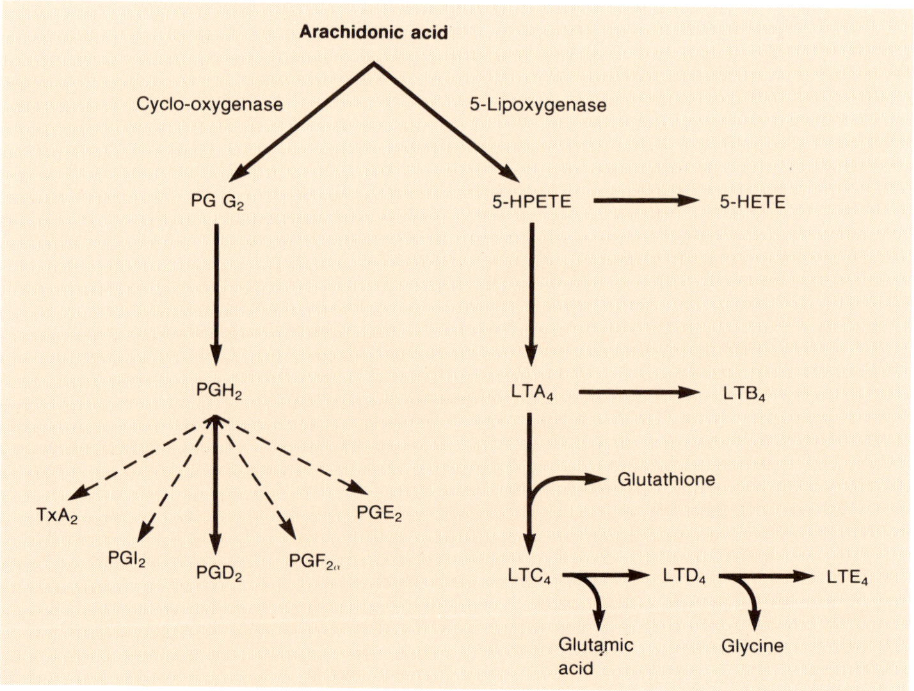

Fig. 1.3. The oxidative metabolism of arachidonic acid by the cyclo-oxygenase and lipoxygenase pathways.

Table 1.1. Classification of non-steroidal anti-inflammatory drugs and their availability in the USA and the UK

Drug	Availability	
	USA	UK
Salicylates and derivatives		
Aspirin in various forms	x	x
Choline magnesium trisalicylate	x	x
Salsalate	x	x
Diflunisal	x	x
Anthranilic acids (fenamates)		
Mefenamic acid	x	x
Meclofenamate sodium	x	
Flufenamic acid		x
Arylacetic acids		
Diclofenac		x
Fenclofenac		w[a]
Arylpropionic acids		
Ibuprofen	x	x
Flurbiprofen		x
Ketoprofen		x
Naproxen	x	x
Fenoprofen	x	x
Fenbufen		x
Indoprofen		w[a]
Tiaprofenic acid		x
Heteraryl acetic acids		
Tolmetin	x	x
Zomepirac	w[a]	w[a]
Indole and indene acetic acids		
Indomethacin	x	x
Sulindac	x	x
Pyrazolidinediones		
Phenylbutazone	x	w[b]
Oxyphenbutazone	x	w[a]
Azapropazone		x
Feprazone		w[a]
Oxicams		
Piroxicam	x	x

a Withdrawn from the market.
b Withdrawn except for treatment of ankylosing spondylitis in patients under hospital care.

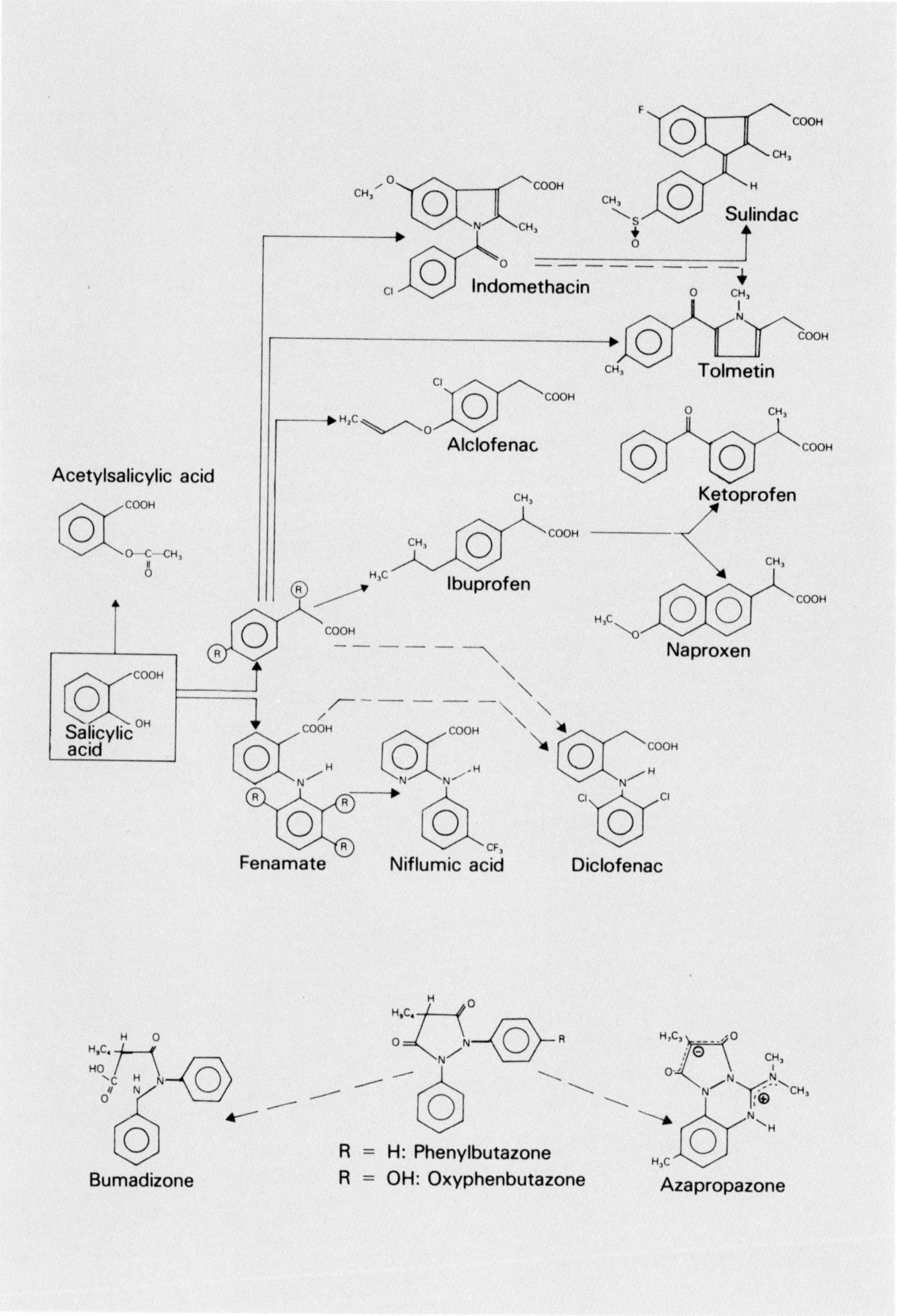

Fig. 1.4. Structural formulae and inter-relationships of some non-steroidal anti-inflammatory analgesics [after Hart, F.D.: Drug Treatment of the Rheumatic Diseases, 2nd ed., p.8 (ADIS Press, Sydney 1982)].

catalyzes the conversion of arachidonic acid to 5-HETE and the leukotrienes. Since 5-HETE and the leukotrienes are also potential mediators of inflammation, a truly effective NSAID would have to inhibit both the cyclo-oxygenase and lipoxygenase pathways (see chapter 5).

Most of the available drugs inhibit only the cyclo-oxygenase pathway and it may be for this reason that they are not entirely effective. The one NSAID which was thought to be an inhibitor of the lipoxygenase pathway, benoxaprofen, is no longer available for clinical use.

Since the prostaglandin system also regulates many other body functions, many of the side effects of the NSAIDs are the direct result of the physiological effect of blocking prostaglandin synthesis. For example, prostaglandins have an effect in controlling renal blood flow – especially in circumstances where there might otherwise be a diminution in blood supply to the kidney. Thus, in certain patients with hypovolemia or other disease processes, inhibition of this regulatory mechanism with an NSAID can result in reduced renal blood flow and decreased glomerulofiltration with subsequent azotemia. Prostaglandins also influence gastric acid production and some of the gastrointestinal toxicity seen with NSAID therapy may result from interference with this system (see chapters 3 and 4).

Classification

The principal NSAIDs now in clinical use – both in the United States and elsewhere – are shown in table 1.1 classified according to their chemical nature, and the structural formulae of some in figure 1.4.

One might think that if a drug in one category were ineffective all the drugs in that category might be ineffective, or that if a patient had a toxic reaction to one, such as a propionic acid derivative, he should then avoid taking all propionic acid derivatives. So far this has not been shown to be the case. However, if the patient is allergic to say a propionic acid derivative, one still might prefer to try an indole or phenylacetic acid or pyrazole derivative rather than another propionic acid derivative despite the fact that use of another drug in the offending class may not provoke a reaction.

Drug Selection

The availability of so many NSAIDs, our limited understanding of their mode of action, and our failure to correlate such characteristics as chemical structure or pharmacokinetic properties with efficacy and tolerance in any consistent way, challenge the prescriber. By examining in more detail factors which might influence the choice of one NSAID rather than another this book attempts, if not to offer a solution, at least to help us order our thoughts on the subject.

2. Clinical Efficacy

Alastair G. Mowat

University of Oxford, Oxford, England

The introduction into clinical practice of a new non-steroidal anti-inflammatory drug (NSAID) has become increasingly difficult both for the manufacturer and the clinician, whether specialist or general practitioner.

Although a different range of NSAIDs is available in different countries (see chapter I) reflecting such factors as the potential market-based upon disease incidence and awareness, the presence of competitive drugs, the demands of the regulatory authorities and the cost-increasingly, clinical and marketing experience in one country is affecting decisions in another. Thus, over recent years, although the development of new NSAIDs has continued unabated, there has been growing delay in their introduction in some countries while several drugs have been withdrawn worldwide after only limited experience of adverse reactions in one country.

Although some of these decisions by regulatory authorities reflect genuine problems with the drugs, there is little doubt that bad prescribing practices, perhaps fuelled by inaccurate advertising, have enhanced the difficulties and may have led to the withdrawal of potentially useful drugs.

It is easy to assume that an NSAID, freely available on prescription, is effective and safe and that its use requires no special consideration by patients or doctor. This chapter examines some of the information required before such assumptions can be made, and attempts to direct the reader of clinical trial reports to potential sources of erroneous results (Kraag, 1982).

The Place of NSAIDs in the Treatment of Arthritic Disorders

Rather than simply accepting the symptoms and disability of arthritic disorders, doctors and patients, with the advent of NSAIDs, have become more aware of treatment possibilities (Wood, 1977). Manufacturers also are aware of the therapeutic and marketing potential for NSAIDs, rheumatic complaints accounting as they do for one-third of attendances at general practitioners' offices and comprising a large number of specialist referrals – a reflection partly of disease frequency and patient demand and partly the relative lack of confidence in diagnosis and treatment, itself a hangover from poor medical school education (McDuffie, 1980). In addition there has been increasing interest in the use of NSAIDs for the treatment of soft tissue injuries, particularly sports injuries and some, e.g. naproxen and naproxen sodium with its rapid onset of action, have been particularly aimed at such patients.

Unfortunately patients' needs and demands, often emphasized in the medical and popular press and tending to center on NSAID therapy, cannot be met. The complexity and severity of some rheumatic diseases means that non-drug therapy, including help and advice from the paramedical team and orthopedic surgery, is also essential for a satisfactory outcome. Furthermore, the natural purpose of the underlying painful, inflammatory condition is to enforce rest and promote healing. Thus, for either doctors or patients to expect total control of symptoms with NSAIDs is unrealistic. Indeed it is important to appreciate that the understanding and expectations of both doctors and patients may be quite different. Hence, the first step in the selection of an NSAID inevitably involves both education and compromise (Potts et al., 1984).

The Inflammatory Process

Unreal expectations of NSAID therapy go hand in hand with our ignorance of the complexity of the inflammatory process and the potential mechanisms of action of these drugs. Despite the apparent diversity of rheumatic and arthritic disorders, a certain uniformity in the early inflammatory process can be assumed. Thus, a variety of triggers, including crystals, bacteria, immune complexes and tissue breakdown products, can all act upon a cell wall, principally that of the neutrophil, to cause activation of the complement cascade and the release of a range of mediators of inflammation including histamine, serotonin, kinins, neutral proteases, superoxide and related radicals and prostaglandins (fig. 2.1). These mediators will cause pain, initiate a number of cellular interactions and tend to perpetuate the inflammatory process which may eventually lead to permanent joint or tissue damage.

Any discussion of the action of NSAIDs tends to emphasize their effect upon prostaglandin production, detracting from the inflammatory potential of the other mediators. The relative inhibitory effect on prostaglandin synthesis in some *in vitro* system is sometimes presented as a reliable measure of a drug's efficacy. The presence of natural inhibitors whether of prostaglandins or other mediators may be ignored. Thus, little attention is paid to caeruloplasmin-inhibiting superoxide and other radicals or the controlling effect of α_1-antitrypsin and α_2-macroglobulin on neutral proteases such as collagenase. At the same time the emphasis on prostaglandin inhibition by NSAIDs ignores their lack of effect upon the lipoxygenase pathway of arachidonic acid metabolism which leads to the production of equally damaging chemicals, superoxide radicals and the leukotrienes (fig. 2.2). To expect that modulation of the activity of a single mediator would have a dramatic effect upon a process of such complexity is illogical and disappointment might have been anticipated by the failure of antihistamines to modify this type of inflammation.

While in some rheumatic conditions the response may be largely chemical, in others, particularly rheumatoid arthritis and related connective tissue diseases, there are complex cellular and immunologic events leading to chronic inflammation. Clearly the potential sites of action of NSAIDs are numerous and greater attention has recently been given to the inhibitory effects of some

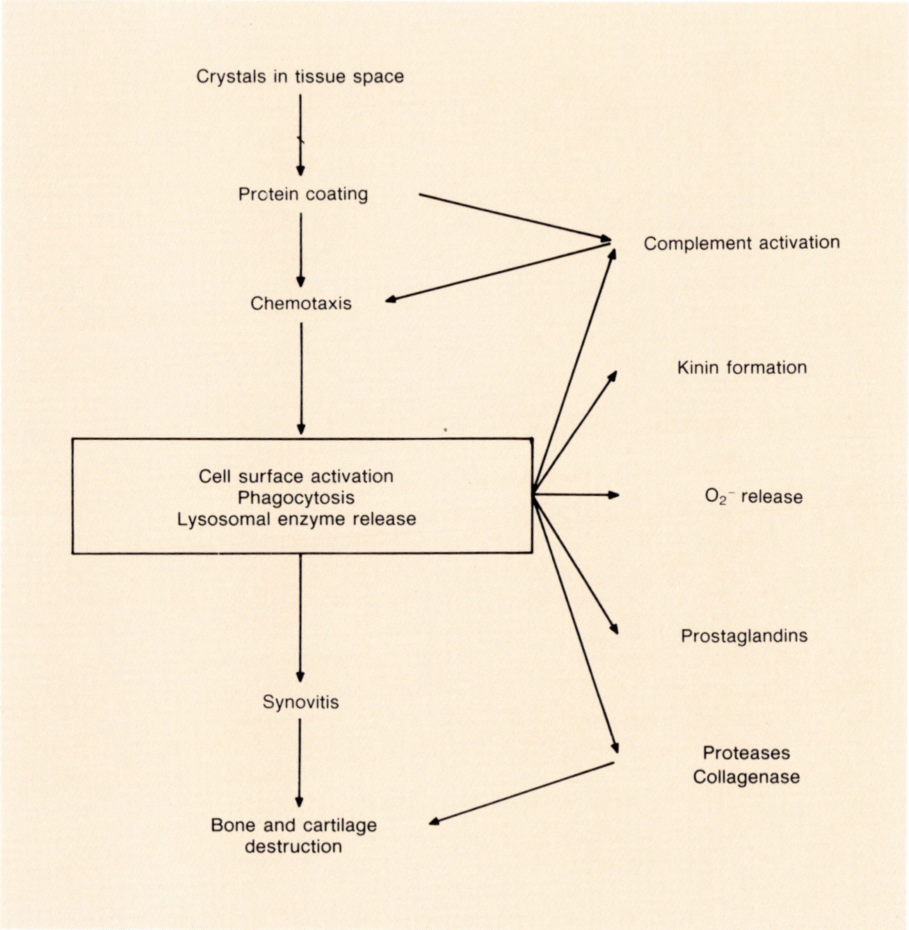

Fig. 2.1. The results of cell activation by foreign material, similar responses being seen for crystals, bacteria, immune complexes and tissue breakdown products.

NSAIDs on immunologically-mediated inflammation. Although it is convenient to examine the effect of a drug on a single chemical reaction in an isolated system using animal cells, this may have little relevance to human disease where there is a range of complementary and competing chemical reactions occurring, some or all of which may be drug-influenced. Also the high protein binding of an NSAID may result in concentrations at the target site that are much lower than those claimed to be effective *in vitro*.

It would be as unwise to assume that all NSAIDs had the same spectrum of activity as it would be to presume that minor differences in inhibition of prostaglandin synthesis were indicative of meaningful differences in clinical efficacy. Hence claims about the importance of an action of an NSAID, particularly a new or unique action, need to be viewed with caution.

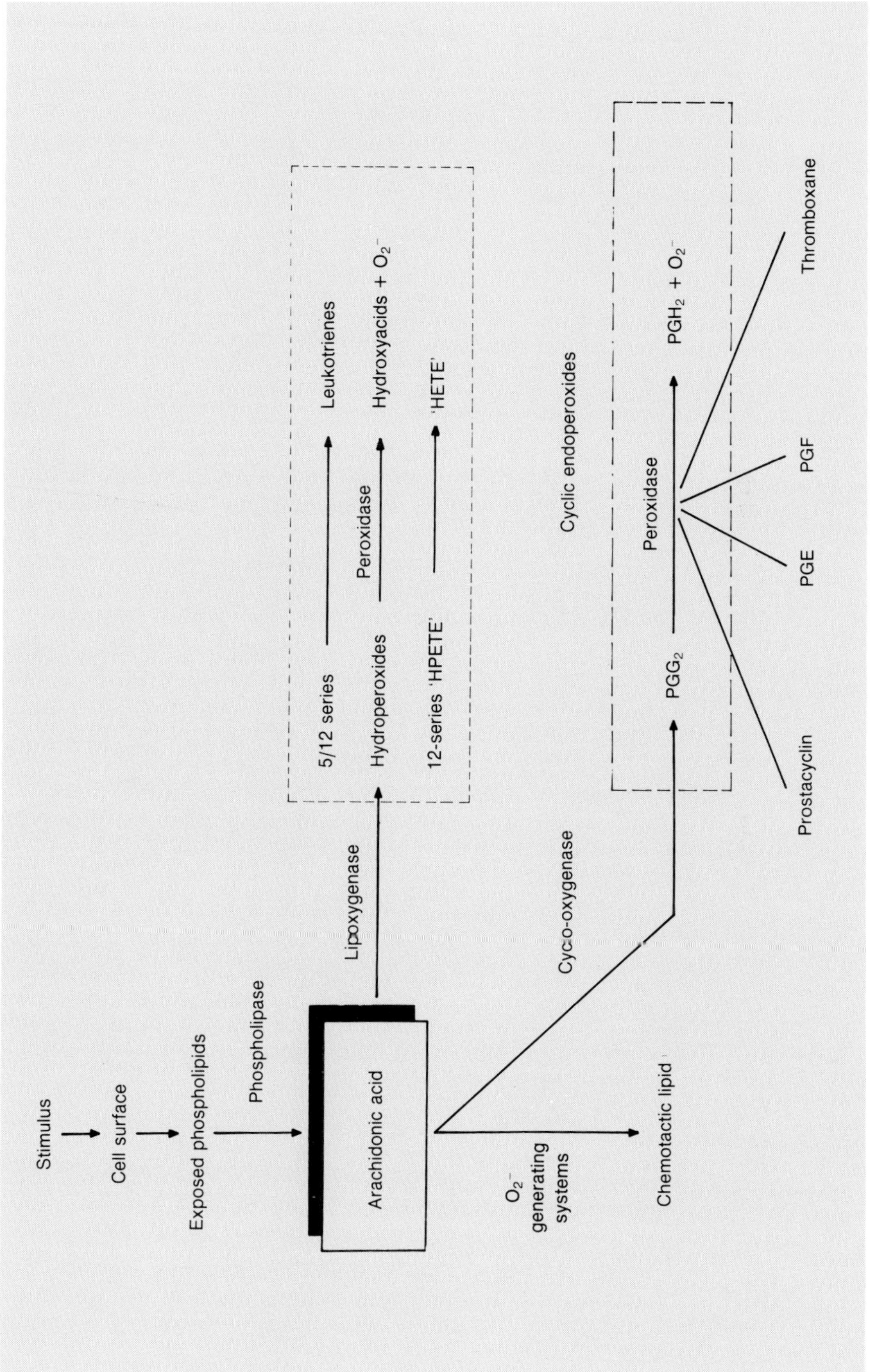

Fig. 2.2. The results of arachidonic acid breakdown.

The Diseases

NSAIDs are widely used to treat arthritic and soft tissue symptoms. Since, as discussed above, the drugs may have different actions in different conditions and perhaps in different patients it is important that treatment groups in clinical trials are homogeneous (Tugwell et al., 1980). This obviously desirable state is not often achieved. The reader should critically examine the clinical status of trial entrants.

Rheumatoid Arthritis

This constitutes the disease group most commonly studied in clinical trials. Using internationally accepted and understood criteria for disease stage, serologic status and simple indicators of disease activity such as erythrocyte sedimentation rate (ESR) and duration of morning stiffness, it should be possible to define a group of patients with early, clinically active and hence potentially controllable disease that is seropositive for rheumatoid factor. All too often trials also include seronegative patients, who may have a different disease (Burns and Calin, 1983), and those with a wide range of disease stages whose capacity to respond may be minimal once the disease process has moved from early inflammatory reaction to late mechanical damage.

The female predominance of the disease (3 : 1) should be reflected in clinical trials. This imbalance between the sexes should not influence drug tolerance as it is well recognized that there is a high incidence of side effects in all rheumatoid patients. This is unexplained, although many feel it must be related to immunologic hyperactivity in these patients (Lyle, 1979).

Ideally patients should be receiving the test drug alone. However, because of difficulties over recruitment and because many rheumatologists feel it may be unethical to withhold slow acting antirheumatic drugs (SAARDs, e.g. gold salts, D-penicillamine) with their potential for disease control, particularly in the early stages, it has become acceptable to include patients whose SAARD or corticosteroid dosage has been unchanged for 3 to 6 months and who are not receiving any local treatment such as physiotherapy or intra-articular injections.

Finally, only outpatients should be included since inpatient treatment, particularly bed rest, can have a significant beneficial effect upon the inflammatory process (Lee et al., 1974).

Osteoarthritis

Definitions for this condition are even looser than for rheumatoid arthritis (Altman et al., 1983). While it may be an end-stage for many different processes it is not necessarily a degenerative process (degenerative joint disease), and some would argue that inflammation is an important etiological component. Certainly this belief encourages the use of NSAIDs rather than analgesics.

Osteoarthritis may be of a variety of types involving single large joints, multiple small joints or the spine, a diversity often ignored when patient groups are selected. Furthermore, as with rheumatoid arthritis, disease staging, which may reflect the inflammatory component and hence the potential response, is usually ignored. The use of patients with a clear disease stage, e.g. those on the waiting list for total hip replacement, often proves unsatisfactory, partly because symptoms are so mechanical and partly because a too favorable response may cause reassessment of the need for a surgical 'cure'.

Finally, the author has found that older patients with single joint osteoarthritis with symptoms clearly related to physical activity are reluctant to become dependent upon drugs and are poorly compliant in clinical trials. Such trials should simulate the female preponderance (2 : 1) and the elderly population. Trials in younger patients who are more easily studied may provide information on only one type of disease, and any extrapolation to the elderly, quite apart from considerations of different drug handling, would be inappropriate. In general a lower incidence of side effects than in rheumatoid arthritis patients can be anticipated.

Other Connective Tissue Diseases

The small number of patients available for study and the complexities of the adjunctive therapy, for instance in systemic lupus erythematosus, mean that little information is generated, although it can be expected that most NSAIDs will be recommended for use in these conditions. Obvious concerns that drugs with a high incidence of skin side effects may prove particularly hazardous in patients with psoriasis or systemic lupus erythematosus have been unfounded. A recent, serendipitous finding that a long-acting preparation of ketoprofen was more effective in psoriatic patients than in rheumatoid arthritis patients may prompt selective trials.

Ankylosing spondylitis is sufficiently common and associated with adequate markers of inflammation such as morning stiffness and measurable spinal and chest movements, that separate trials are undertaken. Once again it is critically important that only those with early, active, potentially improvable disease are included. Even though there is a diagnostic delay of 10 years, the inclusion of patients over the age of 35 is rarely warranted. Men predominate (4 : 1) and this, or other underlying genetic factors not necessarily HLA B27-linked may account for the low incidence of side effects consistently noted in this patient group.

Gout

The short natural history of attacks and the effectiveness of existing NSAID therapy means that few new drugs are tested in patients with gout. Interestingly, despite the tendency to use especially large doses without necessarily a pharmacokinetic basis, there seems to be less interindividual variation of response and a lower incidence of side effects than in rheumatoid arthritis. Thus the failure of a new NSAID to work in acute gout might occasion more interest than its success.

Soft Tissue Lesions

These include a range of conditions in both sporting and non-sporting people, whether intrinsic lesions self-induced by overuse or inappropriate use, e.g. tendonitis or muscle tears, or extrinsic lesions produced by contact, e.g. muscle hematomas. While the necessity to include uniform diagnostic categories and measurements of severity in formal trials can cause difficulties, a greater problem is the establishment of a clinical endpoint in conditions that are self-limiting. Functional testing as well as pain measurement may be employed, while in athletes the return to match fitness is a logical and definable endpoint (Muckle, 1974).

Disease Complexity

It can be postulated that the complexity of an inflammatory process is reflected in the variability of the drug response and the incidence of side effects. Thus gout and soft tissue lesions represent a fairly simple inflammatory process, responsive to most NSAIDs with only modest differences in efficacy and a low incidence of side effects. Ankylosing spondylitis tends to be associated with some differences in drug effect but with a moderate incidence of side effects. Osteoarthritis exhibits increasing complexity with clear interpatient differences, while the intricate inflammation of rheumatoid arthritis is amply matched by differing patient responses and a high incidence of side effects (table 2.1).

Stages in the Development of an NSAID

Animal Studies

A potentially useful new drug emerges only after the screening in animal test systems of many closely related compounds, modified chemically on the basis of known or suspected structure-activity relationships. Modest quantities of carefully purified drug are then given in a variety of doses to small laboratory mammals undergoing standard tests (table 2.2).

Table 2.1. Response to NSAIDs by disease characteristics

Disease	Inflammatory process	Patient preference	Side effects
Soft tissue lesions	Simple	Little	Few
Gout	Simple	Little	Few
Ankylosing spondylitis	Confused	Modest	Occasional
Osteoarthritis	Complicated	Moderate	Frequent
Rheumatoid arthritis	Complex	Great	Multiple

Table 2.2. Standard animal tests for NSAIDs

Anti-inflammatory	
1.	Delay in erythema from ultra-violet light exposure
2.	Reduction in carrageenin-induced paw edema
3.	Reduction in carrageenin-induced pleurisy
4.	Inhibition of the cellular response to subcutaneous sponges
5.	Inhibition of the local, acute and later, systemic phases of adjuvant arthritis in rats
Analgesic	
1.	Reduction in pain in inflamed paws
2.	Reduction in pain in radiant heat test in rat tails
Antipyretic	
Reduced yeast-induced pyrexia	

Further studies of a range of doses of the new drug and existing NSAIDs may suggest order effects and molar potencies that are seldom reflected in clinical practice. At the same time the *in vitro* tests on particular cellular and enzyme systems discussed above (see p.15) may be undertaken, although, in general, they are usually performed later when the new drug's potential attracts the interest of others such as PhD students in the laboratory and other investigators interested in determining the nature of the anti-inflammatory activity of the drug. Lastly, the toxicity data at this stage is crude, simply estimating the single and long term lethal doses, and the type of lesions, including tumors, that may result from long term treatment particularly in the gastrointestinal tract and kidney but rarely including studies of possible teratogenic effects. However, dysmorphogenic studies are routinely performed as investigation of the new drug advances.

In general, the physician should ignore this information which is primarily required by regulatory authorities since it is true that an NSAID that is ineffective in these test systems or extremely toxic in animals is unlikely to be effective or acceptably safe in the treatment of human diseases. The physician should not be deluded by the potency of the new drug relative to that of existing drugs, as any such differences are counterbalanced by final recommended dosages.

Human Studies

Normal Volunteers

A promising drug is now given to human volunteers to define the characteristics of its absorption, metabolism and excretion. Pharmacokinetic studies on single and multiple doses are undertaken so that future patterns of drug prescription in disease can be anticipated. The volunteers are screened for side effects using a wide range of clinical and laboratory parameters. At the same time a number of drug interaction studies are undertaken. Some of the characteristics of these phase I studies are discussed in chapter 5, but it is important for the physician to understand that these are short term studies on small numbers of young, normal, non-diseased individuals and that drug handling may be different in patients.

First Phase of Disease Treatment

Initial phase II studies involve the treatment of a small number of patients with suitable diseases, to confirm that the doses deduced from animal studies are effective and to ensure that the pattern and frequency of side effects are not unexpected. The previously determined data on absorption, metabolism and excretion of single and multiple doses are rarely repeated in these older, diseased individuals.

Ideally, a double-blind comparison with placebo of 2 to 4 weeks' duration using 40 to 60 patients with a single clearly defined active disease should now be undertaken so that realistic clinical, laboratory and side effect data can be generated. It is important that a new drug be demonstrably better than placebo rather than this information be presumed simply because the drug is apparently as effective as another NSAID that has previously been shown to be better than placebo.

Phase II Decisions

At this stage when a major commitment to the drug is being undertaken several serious mistakes can be made.

1. *The wrong dose may be selected.* The history of the NSAIDs abounds with examples of increased dosages being recommended and double-strength tablets being produced within a short time of a drug's introduction. While caution should be applauded, the error has been made so frequently that physicians have come to expect that the dose of all NSAIDs can be (and probably should be) doubled. However, not all enjoy an equal safety margin and there is no substitute for realistic dosage recommendations and sensible warnings about the dangers of exceeding these.

2. *The wrong regimen may be selected.* The absence of pharmacokinetic data in patients may mean the perpetuation of inappropriate dosage regimens. Although ultimately trial and error will determine the best regimen, patient compliance and effectiveness may be compromised by following, for example, a 4-doses-per-day regimen when twice-daily dosage is as effective (Huskisson et al., 1981).

3. *The wrong patients may be selected.* The potential differences in drug handling between the diseased and non-diseased have been alluded to; these differences can be compounded. The elderly and the very young, the two groups who may handle drugs quite differently from healthy young adults, with delayed or accelerated metabolism and excretion respectively (table 2.3), are rarely included in initial studies and thus important differences in efficacy and safety data may be missed. Although subsequent clinical studies are

Table 2.3. The potential results of altered pharmacokinetics in the elderly

Function	Mechanism	Resulting blood level
Absorption	Motility ↓ Mucosal surface ↓	↓
Distribution	Bodyweight ↓ Body water ↓ Body fat ↑ Plasma albumin ↓	↑ Water-soluble drugs ↑ Lipid-soluble drugs ↓ Drug binding ↓ Free drug ↑
Metabolism	Oxidation ↓ Hepatic enzyme induction ↓	↑ ↑
Excretion	Renal function (GFR) ↓	↑

Note: All problems may be compounded by increased drug sensitivity, concomitant disease and polypharmacy with drug interaction and poor compliance.

likely in the young, only recently have the elderly been the subject of formal clinical trials.

By late phase II, the physician should be able to satisfy himself that the drug is clearly better than placebo and that adequate information on dose, regimen and side effects has been generated to ensure the validity of future clinical trials.

Clinical Measurements

In both short and long term clinical trials a variety of measurements are employed. These tend to be expressed in units or to have numerical values attached to them giving the impression that the measurements are absolute, linear, objective and reproducible whereas the very opposite is often the case. Although much the same measurements are employed in most clinical trials this does not necessarily endorse their relevance or value.

Some insight into these measurements will allow non-specialist readers of NSAID trial reports to decide whether the correct parameters have been used, whether the chosen indices and methods of application allow for accuracy and whether it is likely that only small changes and differences, so common in comparative studies of NSAIDs, will be recognized. The scientist lurking within the clinician may overemphasize the objectivity of some measurements while distrusting the subjectivity of others such as stiffness and pain which the physician faces every day in the clinic. Rheumatic symptoms are susceptible to diurnal change and each patient must be seen at the same time at each visit.

Other aspects of trial design, the personnel involved and the number of centers entering patients are considered below.

Duration of Morning Stiffness

Morning stiffness is a diagnostic feature of true inflammation and its duration a measure of disease severity. Although traditionally measured in minutes, most patients find such accuracy impossible. An alternative is to record the presence of stiffness at intervals up to 3 hours using a numerical value even though the record is not truly linear (e.g. 15-minute intervals to 1 hour and then hourly to 3 hours; 1 = less than 15 minutes and 7 = greater than 3 hours). There have been attempts to convert this very subjective stiffness following immobility into a test of function giving more reliable and objective results (Myers et al., 1981).

Pain

Much debate has surrounded the use of either vertical or horizontal visual analog scales for pain, 5-point descriptions of pain and the advisability of patients being presented with the results of earlier tests at the time of recording. None of these scales is linear, the divisions being largely arbitrary. There has perhaps been a swing away from visual analog scales, but there is general agreement that subjective measurements are best and that a reliable, reproducible method, easily understood by patients, must be used to record day and night pain and in osteoarthritis and soft tissue lesions, movement pain.

Finally, it is not pain but pain relief that is being measured. This also is non-linear, it being easier to partly relieve severe pain than to eliminate mild pain. Thus, initial pain scores, and their standard deviation which indicates the number of patients at the two extremes, must be comparable. Occasionally complicated statistics are employed in an attempt to reduce the initial patient differences.

Joint Tenderness and Swelling

A scoring system that records tenderness on pressure, pain on movement, and swelling has been the basis of several indices, the Ritchie Index remaining one of the more reliable measurements of improvement in rheumatoid arthritis. Its responses to firm digital pressure are graded: 0 = no pain, 1 = patient says it is painful, 2 = patient says it is painful and winces, 3 = patient says it is painful, winces and withdraws the limb. Tenderness of the cervical spine, hip, talocalcaneal and midtarsal joints is elicited by passive movement. Some joints such as metacarpophalangeals are treated as units to give a maximum possible score of 78. A similar index more appropriate for osteoarthritis has been described (Doyle et al., 1981). These indices, used by the same experienced observer, are reproducible but remain largely subjective.

Swelling of proximal interphalangeal joints in patients with rheumatoid arthritis has been measured using different instruments for more than 30 years (Hart and Clark, 1951). Provided the patient has early disease with synovial proliferation, and hence swelling that is potentially reducible, the results have proved reliable and objective in the hands of a single observer. These direct joint measurements may show little change in short term trials but with trials of NSAIDs of 8 weeks or more and especially with SAARDs, significant changes, usually recorded as a total for 5 joints per hand, can be expected. Measurements of other joints depend upon a tape measure and have been shown to be poorly reproduced even by a single observer.

Grip Strength

Measured with a modified sphygmomanometer cuff, inflated to 20 or 30mm Hg, the test provides a semi-objective test of hand function reflecting the underlying inflammation and swelling. The test depends upon patient co-operation. Normal individuals can easily record values in excess of 300mm Hg.

Walking Time

The time required to walk a standard distance – 50 feet or 50 metres depending upon clinic facilities – is a semi-objective measurement of lower limb disease since it also depends upon patient co-operation. Recently an attempt has been made to equate preferred walking speeds and their physiologic response to drug effects (Steven et al., 1983).

Joint Movement

Measurement of the range of joint movement, traditionally used by orthopedic surgeons, may show changes with NSAIDs but is inaccurate and time-consuming. Improvement may not reflect useful functional gain, e.g. a knee flexion increase from 120 to 140°.

Measurement of spinal mobility in ankylosing spondylitis, although well researched and apparently responsive to NSAIDs in early disease, does not necessarily reflect changes in the spine measured radiographically (Portek et al., 1983).

Functional Tests

A variety of functional tests have been used, including visual analog scales of certain activities either directed at individual joints, e.g. hip or knee, or personalised to reflect a patient's particular problem with a common function. The latter tests avoid testing function in unaffected joints but more especially eliminate the learning and familiarity phases associated with some unlikely tests devised by therapists, such as hammering in nails (Weintraub et al., 1977).

Radiography and other Physical Measurements

Sequential radiographs of the hands have been used to assess the progress of erosive rheumatoid arthritis. However, the technical difficulties of getting identical pictures, the problem of scoring the lesions, the lag in the emergence of these changes compared with clinical measurements of inflammation and the uncertainty over their variable speed of development means that such radiographs are suitable only for the long term assessment of SAARDs, although they may be used to support claims about the disease-modifying potential of some NSAIDs.

Radioisotope uptake, usually technetium 99^m, xenon clearance, thermography and other methods of measuring skin temperature over a joint, all of which depend upon increased vascularity in and around an inflamed joint, have had their advocates, particularly in rheumatoid arthritis. In general, these methods, although having the attraction of objectivity, are time-consuming and are more appropriate to occasional use over many months in the assessment of SAARDs. They seem to correlate well with clinical measurements.

Laboratory Tests

Laboratory tests have little use in trials of NSAIDs except to monitor potential hepatic, renal and bone marrow toxicity. The erythrocyte sedimentation rate (ESR) and other acute phase reactants, so useful in the assessment of SAARDs, can be expected to show little change even in long term trials of NSAIDs. The hemoglobin will rise and the platelet count fall in parallel with other measurements of decreasing disease activity, but in the short term are more useful as indicators of gastrointestinal blood loss (Farr et al., 1983).

Global Scores

The patient's overall assessment, and to a lesser extent the clinician's overall assessment, has proved to be a useful reflection of a drug's value, combining an appreciation of both the clinical benefits and the side effects. Essentially recorded as a drug being better, the same, or worse than the comparative agent, cumulative, more subtly graded scoring systems have been devised. The close correlation of this very subjective global score with some of the more objective measurements outlined above, has led to its exclusive use in some trials, although the scientist is reluctant to accept such apparently 'soft' and unmeasurable results.

Side Effects

Side effects of NSAIDs are considered in detail in chapters 3 and 4 but clearly have a significant effect upon the ability to measure the results of clinical trials. Withdrawal of a drug because of lack of efficacy or side effects is generally undesirable as it may mask associated side effects or significant clinical benefit respectively and may affect the patient's trust in the clinician's judgement. How much, if any, of the results recorded on patients withdrawn from trials should be used in the final statistical analysis of drug efficacy is a constant cause of concern. Certainly a trial in which there are many withdrawals may be measuring the efficacy of the trial drug in a distinct patient subgroup with characteristics quite different from that of the originally selected study population.

Statistical Analysis

A wide range of statistical methods are employed and the cynic might feel that anything that demonstrates a 'favorable' result is acceptable. In truth, most trials show active drugs to be comparable, but little attention has been focused upon the statistical chance of the trial failing to find a difference, and hence some indication of the numbers of patients and the duration of a trial that would be required to show differences (Buchanan and Smythe, 1982).

Certainly the use of an independent statistician is to be commended as is discussion with the statistician of analytical methods and the numbers of patients required when the trial protocol is being developed. Multivariate analysis, summating the numerical values of several different measurements, has its advocates (Mallya and Mace, 1981) while others favor analysis of covariance which compares a single variable at the end of a trial adjusted for its value at the start.

The striking patient preferences often recorded with NSAIDs naturally leads to close examination of such subsets although it is unusual to find any characteristic that enables their future identification.

Finally, the reader of clinical trial reports must make his or her own judgement as to the *clinical importance* of changes found to be statistically significant.

Comparative Clinical Trials

Short term clinical trials comparing the new drug with established agents and employing the above-mentioned clinical and laboratory measurements constitute late phase II and early phase III in a drug's development. Results of these trials will critically influence the decisions of regulatory bodies and will be the essential information presented to physicians likely to prescribe the new NSAID. Yet the number of potential variables that are all too often hidden in these results and which may invalidate the conclusions are considerable (table 2.4). Those that refer directly to clinical measurements have been considered earlier in this chapter.

Table 2.4. Common design faults of comparative therapeutic trials of NSAIDs

Inadequate number of patients
Non-homogeneous treatment groups
Dosages not equivalent
Inadequate controls to minimize bias and variation
Inappropriate methods of assessment

Disease

The problems of ensuring that a clearly defined and homogeneous population has been treated were discussed on p.18. It is important that the patient group is recognizable to the physician as a sufficiently common entity to make sense of any subsequent treatment proposals. There is clearly a danger, even with a homogeneous disease group, that extrapolation of the data to other patients may be invalid, as is the extrapolation of animal data to humans.

Comparative Drugs

The choice of the comparative drugs, their presentation and dosage regimen are important to the validity of the clinical results. In truth, most investigators who are clinicians actively involved in the field are most anxious to be associated with a trial that offers a valid comparison, the results of which will be respected by their peers. However, the regulatory bodies or the pharmaceutical company providing the comparative drug may place certain constraints on the trial protocol, not recognizing contemporary or changing use of the drug with respect to dose or regimen. The same changing patterns of use may cause unwitting mistakes to be made which become apparent over the 1- to 3-year span between the setting up of the trial and the publication of the results. Despite these complications it is important that the physician's judgement is based upon reasonable comparisons that reflect current clinical usage.

Drug Comparisons

Any NSAID may be used. However, it is only sensible to select a widely used agent, known to be active in the index disease and with an acceptable, predictable incidence and range of side effects. Thus, although aspirin was for many years used as the comparative drug it has been replaced by indomethacin, naproxen or, recently, piroxicam. Tables 2.5 and 2.6 summarize the results of clinical trials in which the efficacy and tolerability of newer NSAIDs were compared with naproxen and indomethacin. Because local factors are becoming increasingly important in drug side effect recognition, ideally the comparative agent should already be available in the country in which the results will be presented.

Dose Comparisons

The daily dose of the comparative drug must be one commonly used. Doses of drugs should not be chosen because of their relative potencies in animal or laboratory test systems; as discussed earlier these may have little relevance to human disease. It is impossible to draw up a list of equipotent daily doses of NSAIDs that enjoys universal agreement. The changing pattern of clinical use and the prescribing habits of the cautious or the cavalier will confound. Yet we all recognize the choice of dose that is sensible and honest. Some argue against fixed doses, claiming that outside clinical trials drug dosages are adjusted initially for patient age and weight and subsequently in line with response and side effects.

Although it is possible to allow patients to adjust drug doses up to certain maximums during the early part of a trial, such doses should then be maintained for realistic clinical and side effect information to be generated (Gall et al., 1982). Variable doses imply a certainty that there is a dose-response curve or a definite age-related factor, neither of which has been clearly demonstrated for most NSAIDs.

Drug Presentation

The presentation of the comparative drug must be that generally used. The requirements of double-blind trials sometimes mean that tablets become capsules or vice versa or that an unprotected form of the drug is used. If such changes are unavoidable it is important that the bioavailability and pharmacokinetics of the new form in diseased patients are properly examined and that changes have not occurred, e.g. in enteric-coating, that make significant changes in pharmacologic or side effect profiles.

Side Effect Profiles

The choice of comparative drug should recognize the expected side effect profiles of both drugs. The number, type and severity of side effects are all important. High dose, unprotected aspirin is easily encapsulated as a comparative trial drug but it is not used in this form in clinical practice due to the high incidence of side effects. Indomethacin is associated with a significant incidence of central nervous system side effects, headache, dizziness, and depression (see tables 2.5 and 2.6), that is well recognized and allowed for in its clinical usage. While it is of considerable interest to know whether the new drug causes similar side effects, when counting total side effects there is no merit in comparing the effects in different body systems. Standard methods of reducing side effects, particularly gastrointestinal effects by taking the drugs with food, must be adopted unless this is known to significantly alter the pharmacokinetics of the agent (see chapter 5).

Table 2.5. The efficacy of the newer NSAIDs in comparison with (a) indomethacin and (b) naproxen: A summary of clinical trials in rheumatoid arthritis

Drug	No. of studies	Anti-inflammatory effect	Analgesia	Side effects	References
a) Indomethacin					
Alclofenac	2	Alc = Ind[a] 2 studies	Alc = Ind 2 studies	Alc = Ind 2 studies (Indomethacin produced more GI disturbance and alclofenac more skin rash)	Brogden et al. (1977)
Carprofen	5	Car = Ind 5 studies	Car = Ind 5 studies	Car = Ind[b] 4 studies (GI disturbances more common with indomethacin; skin reactions more common with carprofen)	Jalava (1983); Kirchheiner et al. (1980); Jensen et al. (1980)
				Car > Ind[c] 1 study	Lussier et al. (1980); Standel (1982)
Diclofenac	10	Dic = Ind 10 studies	Dic = Ind 10 studies	Ind = Dic 8 studies Ind > Dic 2 studies (In general, indomethacin caused more GI and CNS disturbance than diclofenac)	Brogden et al. (1980)
Fenbufen	6	Fen = Ind 4 studies Fen > Ind 2 studies	Fen = Ind 4 studies Fen > Ind 2 studies	Fen = Ind 3 studies Ind > Fen 3 studies	Brogden et al. (1981)
Flurbiprofen	7	Flu = Ind 7 studies	Flu = Ind 7 studies	Flu = Ind 7 studies	Brogden et al. (1979)
Ketoprofen	1	Ket = Ind	Ket = Ind	Ind > Ket	Brogden et al. (1974)
Naproxen	4	Nap = Ind 3 studies Nap > Ind 1 study	Nap = Ind 4 studies	Nap = Ind 1 study Ind > Nap 3 studies	Brogden et al. (1975)

Table 2.5. (contd).

Drug	No. of studies	Anti-inflammatory effect	Analgesia	Side effects	References
Piroxicam	5	Pir = Ind 4 studies Pir > Ind 1 study	Pir = Ind 5 studies	Pir = Ind 4 studies Ind > Pir 1 study	Brogden et al. (1983)
Tolmetin	4	Tol = Ind 4 studies	Tol = Ind 4 studies	Tol = Ind (in 1 study CNS effects were significantly more frequent with tolmetin)	Brogden et al. (1978)
b) Naproxen					
Diclofenac	1	Dic = Nap	Dic = Nap	Dic = Nap	Brogden et al. (1980)
Fenbufen	2	Fen = Nap 2 studies	Fen = Nap 2 studies	Fen = Nap 1 study Nap > Fen 1 study	Brogden et al. (1981) Khan (1983)
Isoxicam	1	Iso = Nap	Iso = Nap	Iso = Nap	Kogstad (1984)
Piroxicam	3	Pir = Nap 3 studies	Pir = Nap 3 studies	Pir = Nap 3 studies	Brogden et al. (1984)
Sulindac	1	Sul = Nap	Sul = Nap	Sul = Nap	Lizarazo and Cortes (1983)

a Alc = Ind indicates results were similar or were not significantly different; Ind > Dic indicates that the first drug was significantly more effective than the second.

b Concern has been expressed regarding the increasing frequency of laboratory signs of liver dysfunction with carprofen (Stein et al., 1983; Wittenberg and Wilmowsky, 1982).

c Car > Ind indicates that adverse reactions were significantly more common with the first drug; Car = Ind indicates that the incidence of side effects was similar or not significantly different.

Regimens

Ideally the daily regimen should conform with that used in clinical practice but the requirements of double-blind trials can make this difficult. Differences, such as twice- or 4-times-daily dosage, may be accommodated by giving matching placebo for the twice-daily drug at the other intervals but this can be interpreted as altering likely patient compliance and hence trial results. Similarly it is not always practical to simulate differential dosing, e.g. small doses of indomethacin 2 or 3 times per day and a large night-time dose.

Table 2.6 The efficacy of the newer NSAIDs in comparison with (a) indomethacin and (b) naproxen: A summary of clinical trials in osteoarthritis

Drug	No. of studies	Overall improvement	Analgesia	Side effects	References
a) Indomethacin					
Alclofenac	3	Alc = Ind[a] 2 studies	Alc = Ind 2 studies Alc > Ind 1 study	Alc = Ind[b] 3 studies	Brogden et al. (1977)
Diclofenac	9	Dic = Ind 8 studies Dic > Ind 1 study	Dic = Ind 7 studies Dic > Ind 1 study	Dic = Ind 8 studies Ind > Dic 1 study (Indomethacin tended to cause more CNS effects)	Brogden et al. (1980)
Fenbufen	3	Fen = Ind 3 studies	Fen = Ind 3 studies	Fen = Ind 2 studies Ind > Fen 1 study	Brogden et al. (1981)
Flurbiprofen	4	Flu = Ind 4 studies	Flu = Ind 4 studies	Flu = Ind 4 studies	Brogden et al. (1979)
Isoxicam	1	Iso = Ind	Iso = Ind	Iso = Ind	Eberl (1982)
Ketoprofen	1		Ket = Ind	Ind > Ket	Brogden et al. (1974)
Piroxicam	3	Pir = Ind 3 studies	Pir = Ind 3 studies	Pir = Ind 2 studies Ind > Pir 1 study (Indomethacin caused significantly more CNS effects; piroxicam caused significantly more skin reactions)	Brogden et al. (1984)
b) Naproxen					
Diclofenac	4	Dic = Nap 3 studies	Dic = Nap 3 studies Dic > Nap 1 study	Dic = Nap 4 studies	Brogden et al. (1980)
Flurbiprofen	1	Flu = Nap	Flu = Nap	Flu > Nap	Brogden et al. (1979)
Isoxicam	1	Iso > Nap	Iso = Nap	Iso = Nap	Turi et al. (1983)

Table 2.6 (contd).

Drug	No. of studies	Overall improvement	Analgesia	Side effects	References
Piroxicam	3	Pir = Nap 1 study Pir > Nap 2 studies	Pir = Nap 3 studies	Pir = Nap 3 studies	Brodgen et al. (1984)

a Alc = Ind indicates that the results were similar or not significantly different; Dic > Ind indicates that the first drug was significantly more effective than the second.

b Alc = Inc indicates that the incidence of side effects was similar or not significantly different; Ind > Dic indicates that significantly more side effects occurred with the first drug.

Trial Duration

Clinical trials can be of different durations depending upon the question that is to be answered.

Very Short Term Trials

These will answer questions of efficacy, with side effects, drug and disease interactions and compliance being largely ignored. Thus, the analgesic effect of NSAIDs on postoperative, dental or osteoarthritic joint pain can be determined over 4 to 6 hours and the initial anti-inflammatory effect over 4 to 7 days depending upon the drug's half-life. However, if such short intervals are to be used, either an educated patient group must be used, who are very familiar with the trial techniques and expected responses, or an additional placebo group must be introduced as the placebo response is likely to be high over this time scale.

Medium Term Trials

Studies of a few weeks' duration will reduce placebo responsiveness enabling a clear pattern of efficacy to emerge; some disease and drug interactions and the commoner side effects should be detected while not compromising compliance in patients who are conscious that they are under close supervision and are anxious to please their physicians. Most consider 4 weeks the optimum time, remembering that although an extended trial may produce more side effect information, the progressive loss of patients due to lack of efficacy and side effects influences the number of patients who must be entered in the trial and the statistical analyses.

Long Term Studies

Trials of several months' or years' duration can demonstrate the continuing efficacy of an NSAID, the possible emergence of a second action, e.g. a disease-modifying effect in rheumatoid arthritis (Berry et al., 1980) or a uricosuric action in patients with gout (Gibson et al., 1984) and the changing pattern of side effects.

In general, since the efficacy of the drug has been established in earlier studies, most of these trials are open and not comparative. Some are conducted by clinicians in special clinics who continue to employ the standard clinical and laboratory measurements to ensure that the drug continues to act. Patients often question whether their system gets used to a drug and whether a change would be sensible. There is no good evidence of the development of tolerance to an NSAID although it might be expected if the underlying inflammatory process had subtly shifted in emphasis so exposing the need for another drug action not provided by the present medication (see p.38).

Furthermore, with increasing length of a trial and decreasing attendance at special clinics the critical factor of patient global assessment may become out of step with other measurements of disease activity. There is value in substantial groups of patients with clearly defined disease being followed in this fairly sophisticated manner to ensure that the number of patient withdrawals due to lack of efficacy and/or side effects is acceptable. Clearly, as discussed earlier, in rheumatoid arthritis it is important that changes in the character of the disease do not make the unchanging character of the therapy unethical. Such studies suggest that at best in a 1-year trial half the patients will continue on the drug (Capell et al., 1979).

Similar trials are required to show whether the drug has a more specific action. Although they are by definition NSAIDs, a slow-acting, antirheumatoid action has been claimed for alclofenac and fenclofenac, both now withdrawn in the United Kingdom. Also, there was limited evidence before benoxaprofen was withdrawn that it too might alter disease course, thus raising the question whether such drugs are bound to have side effect profiles unacceptable for mere NSAIDs. Such SAARD-like action may be unexpected but unless clinical trials, preferably supported by radiographic data, are properly undertaken the opportunity to record unexpected clinical as well as adverse side effects will be missed.

Other trials, usually of 1 to 3 months' duration, are conducted in general practice. They are designed to measure in very simple clinical terms and with crude monitoring of side effects, the drug's performance in the harsh outside world where patient groups are poorly selected, other diseases and treatments are certain to occasionally interact, dissatisfied patients unresponsive to other treatment are likely to be selected for study, compliance may be questionable and the standard of prescribing in respect of existing disease and drugs may be poor (e.g. the patient has a duodenal ulcer and continues taking another NSAID and steroids). Although large numbers of patients may be included, the validity of information produced by such trials may be questioned (Rooney et al., 1978). Attempts to produce more reliable information without improving the other failings in the trials may prove to be self-defeating since the easiest things for patients to claim and for doctors to record are side effects. This is particularly true when there is a climate of distrust about new drugs, and NSAIDs in particular, as occurred in the United Kingdom in the wake of the withdrawal of benoxaprofen in the summer of 1982.

Trial Characteristics

Apart from obvious considerations of patients, drugs and duration, some other factors of comparative clinical trials should be considered as they may influence value judgements.

Who Has Done the Study?

Most of us are happy to accept the results of trials undertaken by clinicians we know and respect. Nationalism may color our judgement about some trials but increasingly such nationalism is being demonstrated by regulatory bodies, often in response to local pressure, with demands that new clinical trials are performed by local physicians on local patients before the overseas data are acceptable as additional evidence. Unfortunately, the move is away from a few well-conducted trials of large numbers of patients in one country to a plethora of small, expensive and increasingly unreliable trials performed by inexperienced physicians in many countries. While there may be national or regional differences in how patients respond to a drug, there is little evidence that current trial techniques are sufficiently sensitive to allow their detection while other factors in trial design and patient selection probably have a greater influence upon results.

This author questions the results of any trial undertaken entirely by busy doctors who rarely have the time and patience to devote to these often boring, repetitive studies on anxious patients whose physical disabilities do not allow them to be hurried. It is vital that this work is delegated to committed professional metrologists who are experienced in trial design, understand measurement of variables, are consistent in the elucidation of side effects, have no preconception of the trial results and have the necessary patience. Senior nurses and physiotherapists are ideal.

One Center or Many?

Ideally these trials should be undertaken at a single center with a single metrologist. Multicenter studies which are sometimes necessary for the enrolment of adequate numbers of patients in a short time are exposed to all the weaknesses mentioned above; no two observers will be the same. While it may be possible by using strict entry and exclusion criteria to enrol similar patients in several centers, the inter-observer differences in most of the clinical measurements, even with experienced metrologists, are considerable. Further, the personal approach, encouragement and enthusiasm of the metrologist will profoundly affect the patient's willingness to persevere with the trial in the face of side effects and lack of efficacy. The statistical analysis of multicenter trials should at least acknowledge and attempt to measure intercenter differences even if some overall conclusions are possible.

Trial Design

Statisticians continue to argue over the merits of crossover or parallel studies. The variability of rheumatic disease probably makes the crossover design, once favored as it seemed to allow direct comparison, less attractive. There are problems in referring back to baseline values in the second treatment period and there may be treatment order effects. Parallel studies demand even closer attention to patient diagnosis and selection.

All studies should be preceded by a drug washout period when only short-acting analgesics are permitted. It is usually impossible to persuade patients with active disease to be without effective drugs for more than 3 days and hence the successful use of longer washout periods questions the selection of patients. It is even more difficult to persuade patients in a crossover trial to follow the ideal format of a second washout between drugs. Since patients may cheat and invalidate this second baseline its use should be examined carefully and a statistical comparison of the 2 baseline indices included in the results.

Practical Drug Usage

Enough has been said about the difficulties and pitfalls of drug development, dosage selection and interpretation of clinical trials to make a cynic of the intelligent physician who is prepared to read some of the literature associated with the introduction of an NSAID. It might be argued that it is easier to continue prescribing existing drugs whose activity is proven, whose side effects are known, whose dosage is established and whose cost is low. Nevertheless, since someone has to provide this information on the new drug and since there is always an element of learning for ourselves the best way to use a drug, some sensible steps can be taken.

As discussed in the introduction we must be conscious of our prescribing habits to try and ensure that drugs are used safely and to the best advantage or we run the risk not only of seeing fewer new drugs but of losing more of those which are now available.

Drug Literature

Drug literature should be examined against the background of problems with clinical trials described above to assess the reliability of the information, the probable clinical benefits in definable patient groups and the type and incidence of side effects. Exotic claims based upon animal experiments should be ignored. Brogden and his colleagues have reviewed the published literature on a number of NSAIDs at intervals over recent years. Their overall conclusions, in terms of efficacy, for several of these drugs are included in tables 2.5 and 2.6. These agree with the generally held view that as a group the newer NSAIDs tend to be as effective as aspirin and indomethacin in formal studies and differences between individual members of the group are not marked.

Patient Selection

It is important that the appropriate patients are chosen for the initial use of a new NSAID. Patients selected should clearly fit one of the diagnoses recommended for treatment and their symptoms and signs should be of sufficient severity to allow some measurement so that patient preferences are not overemphasized. Patients should not continue taking other NSAIDs, or have other diseases under treatment. It is unwise, although tempting, to include patients with a long history of intolerance to NSAIDs or secondary conditions such as peptic ulcers which are known to cause problems with these drugs. 'Difficult-to-treat' patients are almost certain to remain so and the drug's image may be unreasonably tarnished.

Patient Education

Patients must understand the likely benefits and possible side effects of treatment. It is unrealistic to expect the removal of all pain and stiffness, a perfect night's sleep and striking improvement in functional capacity. Patients need to be educated to understand their diseases; measuring gain rather than expecting cure. For most patients with chronic rheumatic diseases, drug therapy is only a part of the overall care and the help and counselling of community-based paramedical workers, physio- and occupational therapists, psychologists, specialist physicians and orthopedic surgeons may be needed.

Drug Regimen and Dosage

The clinical trials will have suggested effective regimens and dosages. While these can be interpreted with some flexibility, common sense should always be applied. Thus, unless there is evidence of pharmacokinetic interaction, NSAIDs should always be taken with food. Most NSAIDs are best taken in at least 2 divided doses daily, usually with the larger dose being taken in the evening to control night-time symptoms and to relieve morning stiffness. Some experimentation with an educated patient is likely to achieve success and hence compliance.

Although it is often presumed that the convenience of once-daily medication is important in drug compliance this may have less relevance in a painful condition when most patients like access to a drug with a discernibly rapid onset of action more than once in 24 hours (Mowat et al., 1984).

With variable kinetics bodyweight is not necessarily a good guide to dosage. Since it is impractical to measure plasma concentrations of any drug but salicylate the NSAID should be given with caution to underweight individuals and should not be given to children or the elderly unless pharmacokinetic and tolerability information on these groups has been generated in the clinical trials. The trend with the safer NSAIDs has been to higher doses matched by double-strength tablets or capsules usually with no increase in side effects (Mowat et al., 1984). However, the safety of this trend should not be anticipated for all products (e.g. piroxicam) and certainly not for a new drug. The wide therapeutic range enjoyed by some drugs is not shared by all, e.g. benoxaprofen (Editorial, 1982). Drug doses should be increased cautiously in patients already showing some response. In the absence of clinical trials indicating a dose-response effect, the use of high doses in an attempt to force disease response is unwise. The logical and progressive increase in NSAID dose, the comparison with other drugs, the use of different regimens and the introduction of new preparations is shown in table 2.6 using naproxen as the example.

Duration of Treatment

In considering the optimum treatment duration for a new drug, much the same considerations apply as in a clinical trial. With a well-educated and experienced patient it may be possible to come to a conclusion in a week but with most, treatment should be continued for 3 to 4 weeks before being abandoned.

There is no rationale for altering the drug dose or regimen if a patient's symptoms are well controlled. Nevertheless, it is important that the patient's condition is periodically re-evaluated, particularly if the diagnosis is rheumatoid arthritis or a related connective tissue disease. Symptom control may not mean disease control and evidence of continuing synovitis and/or radiographic progression should lead to consideration of adding a SAARD. Patients with previously well controlled symptoms of mild, slowly progressive rheumatoid arthritis or osteoarthritis should initially have their dose and/or regimen carefully tailored before the diagnosis is reconsidered and other NSAID therapy started.

As will be discussed in chapter 7 the clinical trial assessment and subsequent clinical usage of NSAIDs is much influenced by individual patient responsiveness and side effects profiles expressed as patient preferences. Effective NSAID therapy should not be abandoned without good cause, while it is equally valid to continue prescribing well tried and effective medication rather than everything new that appears.

References

Altman, R.D.; Meenan, R.F.; Hochberg, M.C.; Bole, G.G.; Brandt, K.; Cooke, T.D.V.; Greenwald, R.A.; Howell, D.S.; Kaplan, D.; Koopman, W.J.; Mainken, H.; Mikkelsen, W.M.; Moskowitz, R. and Sokoloff, L.: An approach to developing criteria for the clinical diagnosis and classification of osteoarthritis. Journal of Rheumatology 10: 180-183 (1983).

Berry, H.; Ford-Hutchinson, A.W.; Camp, A.V.; Heywood, D.; Molloy, M.G.; James, D.W. and Hamilton E.B.D.: Antirheumatic activity of fenclofenac. Annals of the Rheumatic Diseases 39: 473-475 (1980).

Brogden, R.N.; Speight, T.M. and Avery, G.S.: Ketoprofen: A preliminary report of its pharmacological activity and therapeutic efficacy in rheumatic disorders. Drugs 8: 168-175 (1974).

Brogden, R.N.; Pinder, R.M.; Sawyer, P.R.; Speight, T.M. and Avery, G.S.: Naproxen: A review of its pharmacological properties and therapeutic efficacy and use. Drugs 9: 326-363 (1975).

Brogden, R.N.; Heel, R.C.; Speight, T.M. and Avery, G.S.: Alclofenac: A review of its pharmacological properties and therapeutic efficacy in rheumatoid arthritis and allied rheumatic disorders. Drugs 14: 241-259 (1977).

Brogden, R.N.; Heel, R.C.; Speight, T.M. and Avery, G.S.: Tolmetin. A review of its pharmacological properties and therapeutic efficacy in rheumatic diseases. Drugs 15: 429-450 (1978).

Brogden, R.N.; Heel, R.C.; Speight, T.M. and Avery, G.S.: Flurbiprofen: A review of its pharmacological properties and therapeutic use in rheumatic diseases. Drugs 18: 417-438 (1979).

Brogden, R.N.; Heel, R.C.; Pakes, G.E.; Speight, T.M. and Avery, G.S.: Diclofenac sodium: A review of its pharmacological properties and therapeutic use in rheumatic diseases and pain of varying origin. Drugs 20: 24-48 (1980).

Brogden, R.N.; Heel, R.C.; Speight, T.M. and Avery, G.S.: Fenbufen: A review of its pharmacological properties and therapeutic use in rheumatic diseases and acute pain. Drugs 21: 1-22 (1981).

Brogden, R.N.; Heel, R.C.; Speight, T.M. and Avery, G.S.: Piroxicam: A reappraisal of its pharmacology and therapeutic efficacy. Drugs 28: 292-323 (1984).

Buchanan, W.W. and Smythe, H.A.: Can clinicians and statisticians be friends? Journal of Rheumatology 9: 653-654 (1982).

Burns, T.M. and Calin, A.: The hand radiograph as a diagnostic discriminant between seropositive and seronegative 'rheumatoid arthritis': A controlled study. Annals of the Rheumatic Diseases 42: 605-612 (1983).

Capell, H.A.; Rennie, J.A.N.; Rooney, P.J.; Murdoch, R.M.; Hole, D.J.; Dick, W.C. and Buchanan, W.W.: Patient compliance: A novel method of testing non-steroidal anti-inflammatory analgesics in rheumatoid arthritis. Journal of Rheumatology 6: 584-593 (1979).

Doyle, D.V.; Dieppe, P.A.; Scott, J. and Huskisson, E.C.: An articular index for the assessment of osteoarthritis. Annals of the Rheumatic Diseases 40: 75-78 (1981).

Eberl, R.: A double-blind multicenter study comparing isoxicam and indomethacin in the treatment of degenerative joint disease. Seminars in Arthritis and Rheumatism 12: 175-178 (1982).

Editorial: The rise and fall of benoxaprofen. Rheumatology and Rehabilitation 21: 191-192 (1982).

Farr, M.; Scott, D.L.; Constable, T.J.; Hawker, R.J.; Hawkins, C.F. and Stuart, J.: Thrombocytosis of active rheumatoid disease. Annals of the Rheumatic Diseases 42: 545-549 (1983).

Gall, E.P.; Caperton, E.M.; McComb, J.E.; Messner, R.; Multz, C.V.; O'Hanlan, M. and Willkens, R.E.: Clinical comparison of ibuprofen, fenoprofen calcium, naproxen and tolmetin sodium in rheumatoid arthritis. Journal of Rheumatology 9: 402-407 (1982).

Gibson, T.; Simmonds, H.A.; Armstrong, R.D.; Fairbanks, I.D. and Rodgers, A.V.: Azapropazone – a treatment of hyperuricaemia and gout? British Journal of Rheumatology 23: 39-43 (1984).

Hart, F.D. and Clark, C.J.M.: Measurement of digital swelling in rheumatoid arthritis. Lancet 1: 775-776 (1951).

Huskisson, E.C.; Scott, J. and Christophides, N.: How frequently should anti-inflammatory drugs be given? A study with indoprofen. Rheumatology and Rehabilitation 20: 174-176 (1981).

Jalava, S.: A double blind crossover study of carprofen and indomethacin in patients with rheumatoid arthritis. Scandinavian Journal of Rheumatology 48: 5-9 (1983).

Jensen , E.M.; Fossgreen, J.; Kirchheiner, B.; Kryger, J.; Holm, P. and Møllenbach, K.: Treatment of rheumatoid arthritis with carprofen (Imadyl) or indomethacin: A randomized multicentre trial. Current Therapeutic Research 28: 882-887 (1980).

Khan, F.M.: A six-month parallel group comparison of fenbufen and naproxen in the treatment of rheumatoid arthritis. Clinical Therapeutics 5: 483-487 (1983).

Kirchheiner, B.; Fossgreen, J.; Jensen, E.M.; Kryger, J.; Holm, P. and Møllenbach, K.: A new anti-inflammatory agent, carprofen (Imadyl) in rheumatoid arthritis: A randomized multicentre comparison with indomethacin. Current Therapeutic Research 28: 875-881 (1980).

Kogstad, O.: A 4-week parallel group, double-blind comparison of isoxicam 200 mg daily with naproxen 250mg three times daily in patients with rheumatoid arthritis. Scandinavian Journal of Rheumatology (Suppl. 53): 97 (1984).

Kraag, G.R.: The NSAID dilemma – too many or too few? Journal of Rheumatology 9: 655-657 (1982).

Lee, P.; Kennedy, A.C.; Anderson, J. and Buchanan, W.W.: Benefits of hospitalization in rheumatoid arthritis. Quarterly Journal of Medicine 43: 205-214 (1974).

Lizarazo, P.H. and Cortés, M.P.: Single-blind parallel study comparing naproxen with sulindac and with diclofenac in rheumatoid arthritis. Current Therapeutic Research 34: 701-707 (1983).

Lussier, A.; Rouleau, L.; Caron, M. and Tetreault, L.: Comparative evaluation of carprofen and indomethacin in rheumatoid patients. International Journal of Clinical Pharmacology, Therapy and Toxicology 18: 482-487 (1980).

Lyle, W.H.: Penicillamine. Clinics in Rheumatic Diseases 5: 569-601 (1979).

Mallya, R.K. and Mace, B.E.W.: The assessment of disease activity in rheumatoid arthritis using a multivariate analysis. Rheumatology and Rehabilitation 20: 14-17 (1981).

McDuffie, F.C.: The need to train family practitioners in rheumatology. Journal of Rheumatology 7: 772-773 (1980).

Mowat, A.M.; Mowat, A.G.; Jones, C.W. and Engler, C.: A comparison of once and twice daily naproxen in rheumatoid arthritis. British Journal of Clinical Practice 38: 95-98 (1984).
Muckle, D.S.: Comparative study of ibuprofen and aspirin in soft-tissue injuries. Rheumatology and Rehabilitation 13: 141-147 (1974).
Myers, D.B.; Wilson, K. and Palmer, D.G.: An objective measurement of change in morning stiffness. Rheumatology International 1: 135-137 (1981).
Portek, I.; Pearcy, M.J.; Reader, G.P. and Mowat A.G.: Correlation between radiographic and clinical measurement of lumbar spine movement. British Journal of Rheumatology 22: 197-205 (1983).
Potts, M.; Weinberger, M. and Brandt, K.: Views of patients and providers regarding the importance of various aspects of an arthritis treatment programme. Journal of Rheumatology 11: 71-75 (1984).
Rooney, P.; Buchanan, W.W.; Haigh, B.S.; Roylance, P.J. and Rhymer, A.R.: A clinical assessment in general practice of sulindac. European Journal of Rheumatology and Inflammation 1: 66-68 (1978).
Standel, W.: Clinical trials in rheumatoid arthritis. European Journal of Rheumatology and Inflammation 5: 503-506 (1982).
Stein, G.H.; Dickey, R.A. and Cohn, P.D.: Controlled comparison of carprofen and aspirin in osteoarthritis of the knee. Current Therapeutic Research 33: 415-422 (1983).
Steven, M.M.; Capell, H.A.; Sturrock, R.D. and MacGregor, J.: The physiological cost of gait: A new technique for evaluating nonsteroidal anti-inflammatory drugs in rheumatoid arthritis. British Journal of Rheumatology 22: 141-145 (1983).
Tugwell, P.; Sackett, D.L. and Haynes, R.B.: On the critical assessment and clinical applicability of the rheumatology literature. Journal of Rheumatology 7: 765-771 (1980).
Turi, G.; Boscaro, C. and De Bastiani, G.: Double-blind comparative study of isoxicam and naproxen in the treatment of patients with osteoarthritis. Current Therapeutic Research 33: 83-88 (1983).
Weintraub, M.; Jacox, R.F.; Angevine, C.D. and Attwater, E.C.: Piroxicam in rheumatoid arthritis: A controlled clinical trial with novel assessment techniques. Journal of Rheumatology 4: 393-404 (1977).
Wittenborg, A. and Wilmowsky, H.: Carprofen in ankylosing spondylitis. European Journal of Rheumatology and Inflammation 5: 527-535 (1982).
Wood, P.H.N.: The Challenge of Arthritis and Rheumatism (British League Against Rheumatism, London 1977).

Additional Reading

Huskisson, E.C.: Anti-rheumatic drugs. Clinics in Rheumatic Diseases 5: 351-733 (1979).
Huskisson, E.C.: Anti-rheumatic drugs II. Clinics in Rheumatic Diseases 6: 463-695 (1980).
Huskisson, E.C.: Anti-rheumatic drugs III. Clinics in Rheumatic Diseases 10: 217-432 (1984).
Klippel, J.H. and Decker, J.L.: Clinical trials in the rheumatic diseases. Clinics in Rheumatic Diseases 9: 489-695 (1983).
Kirwan, J.R.; Chaput de Saintonge, D.M.; Joyce, C.R.B. and Currey, H.L.F.: Advances in assessing rheumatoid arthritis. British Journal of Rheumatology (Suppl.): (1983).

3. Major Toxic Reactions Associated with NSAIDs

P.D. Fowler

Staffordshire Rheumatology Centre, Stoke-on-Trent, England

Information from the Arthritis Foundation suggests that there are at least 7.5 million people in the United States with rheumatoid arthritis as well as 30 million other sufferers of chronic rheumatic disorders. NSAIDs are the single most commonly prescribed group of drugs; 1 in 7 Americans is at some time likely to be treated with one of them. It is thus not surprising that severe adverse reactions are observed, even when they occur in only 1 per 100,000 patients treated.

The commonest causes for withdrawal of treatment are the relatively minor subjective symptoms such as dyspepsia and heartburn or, less frequently, the minor central nervous system symptoms, headache and dizziness (particularly with indomethacin), diarrhea and skin rashes (see chapter 4). By far the most frequent causes of major morbidity or mortality are gastrointestinal hemorrhage from multiple gastric erosions or ulcer, and perforation of a gastric or duodenal ulcer which has developed while the patient has been taking the drug.

Much more dramatic are the far less frequent complications; blood dyscrasias, florid skin reactions such as erythema multiforme, toxic epidermal necrolysis (Lyell's syndrome) and acute hepatitis. Other potentially fatal reactions include acute hypersensitivity reactions with bronchospasm, cardiac failure following fluid retention and renal impairment.

Difficulties in Identifying Drugs Causing Adverse Reactions

When a patient who is taking only one drug develops an acute reaction such as rash, an idiosyncratic reaction or acute edema shortly after the onset of therapy it is not unreasonable to attribute the complication to the drug. Similarly, if after prolonged therapy with only one drug a chronic peptic ulcer or aplastic anemia occurs, it is reasonable to consider the drug as a likely cause – though both may arise *de novo*.

In practice, however, matters are rarely so simple. Patients, particularly the elderly or those with rheumatoid arthritis, are often taking many drugs. If a drug with a reputation (deserved or otherwise) for causing a particular reaction is part of the treatment regimen this particular preparation will be singled out for blame and so its unfortunate reputation is further emphasized. As an example, a patient with rheumatoid arthritis treated for a prolonged period with aspirin and gold therapy became progressively ill over some months. Treatment was eventually withdrawn and phenylbutazone substituted. One week later aplastic anemia was diagnosed and attributed to the phenylbutazone.

It is rare for the disease being treated to be considered as a contributing factor to a 'drug reaction', yet a simple study (Fowler and Faragher, 1977) has shown that patients with rheumatoid arthritis are, proportionately, much more likely to suffer adverse drug reactions than those with osteoarthritis.

Similarly, racial and genetic factors play their part. In the United Kingdom and many other countries where aspirin compounds are used extensively the drug ibufenac was withdrawn because of hepatic toxicity. In contrast, ibufenac was used extensively for many years without major problems in Japan, where aspirin is very poorly tolerated.

Discrepancies in Reporting

In some countries, national agencies exist for the collection and collation of adverse drug reaction data, such as the Committee on Safety of Medicines in the United Kingdom. This organization does not set out to attribute reactions to a particular compound, however. Its function is to collect reports and recognize the early signs of a potential danger. If a patient develops agranulocytosis while taking say, aspirin, D-penicillamine and a diuretic, the reaction will be recorded in each of three files.

There is a wide divergence of attitude among doctors, depending on the type of adverse reaction. Gastric bleeding or perforation are acknowledged as acceptable risks of NSAID therapy. The incident has a rapid conclusion and the doctor has no feeling of guilt. In contrast, when a patient develops aplastic anemia and the doctor has to treat the patient, perhaps for many months, throughout a most horrible and perhaps eventually fatal illness he may become racked with guilt, particularly if he frequently has to face distressed relatives. This type of reaction will always be reported, and the doctor will probably never use the drug again regardless of its relative merit, even though the final outcome in the examples cited above may be identical.

Reporting Frequency

Weber (1984) has demonstrated a historical cycle of reporting frequency. Studying 7 NSAIDs he showed that the rate of reporting increases, usually towards the end of the second year of marketing, and thereafter declines regardless of the usually increasing prescribing rate.

The length of time since the introduction of a compound has other important effects, as does the early experience with the compound. Many of the more recently marketed preparations were introduced at a very low dosage and so gained a reputation for excellent tolerance and safety: ibuprofen was initially prescribed at a dosage of 200mg tid but is now prescribed at a dosage of 2.4g daily; naproxen used initially at 750mg daily may now be given up to 2.0g daily. In contrast, phenylbutazone was first used in a daily dosage of more than 1g, then 800mg daily was common for many years, but the recommended dosage now is 200 to 300mg daily. Similarly, drugs available for many years now have large dossiers of adverse effect reports. A recent United Kingdom press report noted (incorrectly) that more than 400 deaths had been associated with oxyphenbutazone – but even then did not comment that it had been available for nearly 25 years.

Problem Patients

It has already been noted that patients with certain diseases are more prone to adverse reactions (see also chapter 2, table 2.1). Patients at the extremes of life – infants and the elderly – metabolize some drugs differently and may be particularly at risk, as may other patients with diseases of excretory or metabolizing systems (table 3.1; see also chapter 6).

Non-medical Influences

In recent years the growth of consumerism has resulted in increasing exploitation of adverse drug reactions by press and politicians. Although reputedly protecting the public interest it is done mainly to promote self-interest. The resulting pressures have led to decisions by national drug regulatory bodies that appear to be influenced more by political expedience than medical science, so that worthwhile compounds may have been prematurely withdrawn.

Experience in a Large Rheumatology Unit

The Staffordshire Rheumatology Centre employs 4 senior rheumatologists. The routine outpatient clinic rate is currently 1260 new patients and 7800 follow-up consultations per annum. In addition there are combined clinics with orthopedic and pediatric specialists, 2 members of the team consult outside the National Health Service and during 1983 there were 343 inpatient treatments usually of 2 to 3 weeks' duration. Thus the combined annual consultation rate for the unit is approximately 10,000.

The major disease is rheumatoid arthritis and other variants of inflammatory polyarthritis. Virtually all these patients are taking one NSAID, many are having two, a common combination being a slow-release indomethacin at bedtime (75mg or 100mg suppository) together with naproxen (250mg tid or more) or diclofenac sodium (50mg tid) during the day. These are the most

Table 3.1. Influence of age and disease on the pharmacokinetics of commonly used NSAIDs

	Metabolic handling in					Dosage adjustment	
	infancy and children	old age	active RA	renal failure	hepatic failure	renal	hepatic
Indomethacin	↑↑	0	0	⇡	↑	?	√
Diclofenac sodium	0	0	0	⇡		√[a]	?
Naproxen	0	0		0	↑	0	√
Piroxicam	0	0	0	0	↑	0	√[a]
Ibuprofen and flurbiprofen		0	0	0		√[a]	√[a]
Fenclofenac							
Aspirin and variants	↑↑	↑	0	↑		√	?
Phenylbutazone and oxyphenbutazone	↓	0	0	↑	0	√	√
Azapropazone		↑		↑	↑	√	√
Fenamates		⇡				?	?
Fenoprofen	0	0				0	?
Fenbufen		0		0		0	?
Ketoprofen		↑		↑		√[a]	?

Key to symbols:
↑↑ = Definite marked increase in plasma drug concentration.
↑ = Plasma concentrations increased.
⇡ = Plasma concentrations increased in extreme situations.
↓ = Plasma concentrations decreased.
0 = No effect.
√ = Dosage decrease needed.
a = In extreme impairment only.
? = Data not available to enable definite indication.

frequently used preparations, but piroxicam, fenclofenac, ibuprofen and flurbiprofen are also used. Most of the patients with rheumatoid arthritis have severe disease and many are taking second-line drugs [chloroquine, dapsone, D-penicillamine, gold and salazopyrine (sulphasalazine)] in addition to their NSAID. Systemic corticosteroid therapy is used rarely for uncomplicated rheumatoid arthritis. Safety monitoring of second-line drugs is rigorous.

During the past 5 years, serious adverse drug reactions have been remarkable for their rarity. The majority have been related to gold or D-penicillamine therapy. We have seen numerous skin and/or mucocutaneous reactions to gold, but only 4 patients with severe or protracted eczematous lesions and only one Stevens-Johnson syndrome. This latter resolved in a few months following withdrawal of high dose therapy. Some patients have had low white cell counts but there have been no cases of blood dyscrasias. With penicillamine skin problems have been less troublesome, but 5 or 6 patients have required withdrawal of treatment because of low platelet counts, though none was below 50,000 c/ml. Two have shown low white cell counts. Four cases of heavy albuminuria have occurred; all have recovered. One patient has obliterative bronchiolitis. One patient developed penicillamine-induced lupus erythematosus, and one hypoglobulinemia. We have seen numerous cases of mild hemolytic and macrocytic anemia related to dapsone treatment and a small number with salazopyrine.

In contrast, serious reactions to NSAIDs have been infrequent. There have been 10 to 15 cases of gastrointestinal bleeding or ulcer perforations with indomethacin, and perhaps 20 more of anemia related to gastrointestinal blood loss with other NSAIDs. One patient on gold therapy developed severe hemolytic anemia shortly after commencing piroxicam, one developed renal failure requiring dialysis with benoxaprofen, and one patient developed a severe Stevens-Johnson syndrome while taking diclofenac sodium. Water retention resulting in congestive heart failure has been seen in 3 patients taking indomethacin and 2 or 3 with hypertension have required indomethacin withdrawal before this could be controlled with appropriate drugs.

Which NSAID to Choose? (see also chapter 7)

Although it is of prime importance to be aware of the potential major toxicity with any drug used, it should be clear from the foregoing that, except for the blood dyscrasias associated with phenylbutazone and related compounds, major toxic effects are not a prime consideration when selecting NSAID therapy. Symptomatic intolerance, particularly gastric intolerance, is the greatest problem, especially with indomethacin which is one of the most effective of those in common use. In selecting an NSAID it is perhaps worth emphasizing that some preparations have been in use for many years, particularly aspirin, phenylbutazone and indomethacin, so that their potential toxicity is fully established. Many of the propionic acids, especially naproxen, ibuprofen and ketoprofen, have been available long enough to assume that nothing unexpected will now occur. Two of the more recent arrivals, diclofenac sodium and piroxicam have also been used very extensively.

Before cataloguing the features of individual preparations the age-old advice, which cannot be bettered, is worth repeating. The non-specialist in this field should become totally familiar with and use only 3 or 4 NSAIDs; one which is very powerful if less well tolerated (say indomethacin), another excellently tolerated preparation for difficult patients (perhaps ibuprofen), and 2 very effective and normally well tolerated drugs (say naproxen and diclofenac sodium) should be sufficient in most instances.

Pharmacokinetic Variation in Disease and According to Age

There are a number of situations in which the pharmacokinetic or metabolic handling may be altered and so increase the possibility of drug toxicity (table 3.1; see also chapter 6). Neonates have undeveloped hepatic enzyme systems. Elderly patients may have lower serum proteins and diminished renal function so that higher plasma levels of non-protein-bound drug may be present. Drug handling may be affected by the activity of the inflammatory process, for example higher blood levels of propranolol are seen in patients with active inflammatory disease (Babb et al., 1976).

Because NSAIDs are highly protein-bound and excreted mainly as soluble urinary metabolites it would be expected that renal failure would cause serious problems. In fact, it is only with significant renal disease that problems arise.

Usually, as renal excretion diminishes there is a compensatory increase in biliary excretion. Although hepatic metabolism is important, it is only in the most severe cases of hepatic insufficiency that metabolism is impaired, though detailed studies with individual drugs are rare. A major problem to be expected in these higher risk patients is gastrointestinal hemorrhage.

Specific Major Toxicity

Data available from the Committee on Safety of Medicines (CSM) [1984], as already noted, have to be interpreted with particular care because of variations in reporting levels and the wide variation in the amounts of individual drug usage. Nevertheless, they form one of the very few bases for inter-drug comparisons.

Table 3.2 is prepared from CSM data (Committee on Safety of Medicines, 1984). Because the gross figures make comparisons difficult, annual rates have been calculated, though some of these, as indicated, include reports collected prior to marketing the drug. The table is arbitrarily divided into high, medium and low prescription groups. Nevertheless the table clearly identifies the high blood dyscrasia rate for phenylbutazone and oxyphenbutazone and the obviously high overall toxicity of benoxaprofen. Apart from one or two exceptions such as the increased annual frequency of severe skin reactions with fenbufen, fenclofenac and piroxicam, the reporting rates for this wide range of compounds are remarkable for their similarity.

Included under the heading of hepatic toxicity are the diagnoses hepatic failure, hepatitis and cholestatic jaundice. Listings such as abnormal hepatic function and 'SGOT increased' have been assumed to be liver function test abnormalities and are not included. Only benoxaprofen appears to be outstanding in this listing.

Severe skin reactions include only exfoliative dermatitis, erythema multiforme, toxic epidermal necrolysis, Lyell's syndrome and Stevens-Johnson syndrome. They do not include such diagnoses as rash, erythema, pruritus, etc., which have been assumed (rightly or wrongly) to refer to relatively minor conditions. Again benoxaprofen features in this list, but fenbufen also rates highly, due mostly to reports of erythema multiforme.

Table 3.2. Adverse reaction reports to the UK Committee on Safety of Medicines: estimated rate (fatal rate) per annum

Drug (years available)	Overall rate	Blood dyscrasias[a]			Hepatic reactions[b]	Severe skin reactions[c]
		(i)	(ii)	(iii)		
High prescription-rate drugs						
Phenylbutazone (24)	70 (18)[d]	15.2 (10)	2.7 (1.6)	2.9 (0.8)	2.5 (0.3)	2.9 (0.4)
Oxyphenbutazone (22)	23 (6)	5.6 (3.8)	1.5 (0.5)	1.5 (0.6)	1 (0.05)	0.7 (0.1)
Indomethacin (19)	144 (13)	2.4 (1.1)	0.6 (0.2)	2.8 (0.2)	2.2 (0.5)	0.61
Ibuprofen (15)	82 (2)	0.7 (0.6)	0.5	3.2 (0.1)	1.5 (0.07)	0.6
Naproxen (11)	119 (6)	1.7 (1)	0.7 (0.1)	2.7 (0.3)	1.1 (0.1)	1.4 (0.1)
Diclofenac (5)	178 (3)	0.2 (0.2)		2.8	5.4	3.2
Piroxicam (5)[e]	354 (9)	1.4 (0.8)	0.2	2.4	2.4 (0.2)	8 (0.4)
Benoxaprofen (3)	1321 (28)	6.3 (0.3)	2 (1.3)	12.3 (0.6)	30 (10.6)	16.6 (1.3)
Medium prescription-rate drugs						
Flurbiprofen (7)	124 (2.5)	0.7 (0.4)		1.1	1.4	0.4
Ketoprofen (13)	52 (1.3)	0.3 (0.07)		1.1 (0.07)	0.07	0.4
Fenbufen (5)[e]	462 (1.4)	1.4 (0.2)	0.2	0.6	0.4	13.0
Fenoprofen (10)	42 (2)	1.5 (0.6)	0.1	1.2 (0.1)	0.5 (0.2)	0.4 (0.1)
Fenclofenac (5)[e]	179 (1.2)	0.6	0.2	1.1	2.2	6.2 (0.2)
Azapropazone (9)	93 (2.3)	0.6 (0.1)		0.3 (0.1)	0.6	1.1
Low prescription-rate drugs						
Tiaprofenic acid (3)	86 (1.3)				0.6	0.6
Indoprofen (2)	130 (4)					
Tolmetin (5)[e]	11				0.2	0.2
Feprazone (8)	149 (0.7)	0.21 (0.1)	0.2 (0.2)	1.2	3.2	2.5 (1.2)
Flufenamic acid (15)	6 (0.1)	0.13 (0.1)		0.1	0.07	0.07
Mefenamic acid (20)	36 (1)	0.2 (0.1)	0.1 (0.1)	0.5 (0.1)	0.3 (0.1)	0.7 (0.1)
Diflunisal (7)	112 (1.4)	0.1 (0.1)		1.3	1.4 (0.1)	4.5
Sulindac (7)	77 (1.3)	0.4 (0.1)		1.1	4.1	1 (0.1)
Others						
Aspirin (20)	176 (4.4)	0.05		0.3	0.2 (0.05)	0.05
Benorylate (12)	32 (0.3)				0.2 (0.1)	0.16

a Blood dyscrasias: (i) includes aplastic and hypoplastic anemia, marrow depression and pancytopenia, (ii) is agranulocytosis but excludes 'leukopenia' and granulocytopenia; (iii) thrombocytopenia.

b Hepatic reactions include all forms of hepatitis and jaundice but not liver function test abnormalities.

c Severe skin reactions are exfoliative dermatitis, epidermal necrolysis, erythema multiforme and Stevens-Johnson syndrome.

d Rate of fatalities.

e Duration of availability: reports precede this by some years.

Table 3.3. The frequency of specific blood dyscrasias with various NSAIDs: unranked comparisons (Weber, 1984)

Drug	Approximate no. of prescriptions for one ADR report (thousands)		
	agranulocytosis	pancytopenia	thrombocytopenia
Feprazone[a]	–	–	34
Benoxaprofen[a]	100	550	60
Fenclofenac[a]	69	–	–
Sulindac	644	644	160
Diclofenac	–	–	110
Azapropazone	–	360	180
Flurbiprofen	–	660	220
Diflunisal	1312	–	220
Piroxicam	570	2280	380

a Withdrawn from the market in the UK.

Blood Dyscrasias

Although Weber (1984) evaluated only 9 of the NSAIDs under consideration, his findings are of interest (table 3.3). He studied only the reports in the first 2 years following marketing and ranked these according to the number of prescriptions. He stresses the statistical crudeness of his findings but they are nevertheless valuable in a field notable for a lack of precise data. He found feprazone, benoxaprofen and fenclofenac to be the group with the most frequently reported blood dyscrasias, with one report per 17,000 to 69,000 prescriptions, piroxicam being the least frequent (one per 207,000) and sulindac, diclofenac, azapropazone and flurbiprofen in the intermediate group (one report per 107,000 to 187,000). Taken directly from his report, table 3.3 shows thrombocytopenia reported with all but fenclofenac. Pancytopenia was not reported with fenclofenac and diflunisal, and neither pancytopenia nor agranulocytosis was reported with feprazone and diclofenac.

Phenylbutazone and Oxyphenbutazone

Agranulocytosis, aplastic anemia and thrombocytopenia were first reported in the 1950s shortly after phenylbutazone became generally available for clinical use. In the United Kingdom, phenylbutazone is now available only to treat ankylosing spondylitis in hospital and oxyphenbutazone has been withdrawn. Initially, the dose prescribed was much higher (up to 1.5g per day) than now used, and there were individual reports of horrendous reactions, with agranulocytosis, hepatitis and severe skin reactions sometimes appearing concurrently.

Because of its therapeutic benefits, the recognition of the value of much lower doses with consequently less toxicity, and in the absence of an alternative other than aspirin at the time, phenylbutazone usage increased rapidly. Nevertheless, serious toxic reactions continued to occur. An analysis of 133 blood dyscrasias (Fowler, 1967) demonstrated that agranulocytosis was an acute reaction occurring early in treatment, whereas aplastic anemia developed insidiously only after prolonged therapy. Elderly female patients were particularly at risk.

Using data collected in the United Kingdom up to 1965 and relating this to the number of prescriptions issued, it was estimated that for phenylbutazone there was one blood dyscrasia per 150,000 'patient months' treatment and one fatal case per 250,000 'patient months'. Inman (1977), using a similar technique but tracing cases via death certificates, estimated a rate of 16.6 and 40 deaths per 100,000 'patient years' for phenylbutazone and oxyphenbutazone respectively.

As well as being of the same order as the figures in the earlier work, the finding that elderly females were a high risk group was also confirmed. The higher rate for oxyphenbutazone is partly related to the finding that relatively more patients were treated with shorter courses. Because of the methods used these figures cannot be compared with those given by Weber (1984) for other drugs.

Feprazone and Azapropazone

Feprazone, which has been withdrawn from the market in the United Kingdom because of skin and gastrointestinal effects, has also been associated with blood dyscrasias, but the overall usage has been so much less that one cannot draw detailed conclusions. Blood dycrasias are rare with azapropazone. This may be because there is no circulating hydroxy-metabolite in the plasma.

Indomethacin

Reports of adverse reactions to indomethacin to the United Kingdom Committee on Safety of Medicines, though less frequent than for phenylbutazone, are numerically such that they cannot be dismissed (Girdwood, 1974), especially as they have occurred in patients who had no other drugs (Mason, 1968), and include agranulocytosis, aplastic anemia and thrombocytopenia.

Although figures to estimate frequency are not available, Inman (1977) identified 85 cases when a drug was the 'probable factor'. Of these, 28 related to phenylbutazone, 11 to oxyphenbutazone and 8 to indomethacin. The relative prescription rates were 820,000, 135,000 and 700,000 per quarter.

Propionic Acid Derivatives

Blood dyscrasias are extremely rarely associated with this group of drugs. A case of bone-marrow depression associated with ibuprofen was noted by

Adams and Warwick-Buckler (1983) and Inman (1977) records 4 possible and one probable association. Cases have not been associated with flurbiprofen, but have been noted with benoxaprofen. Naproxen, another extensively used drug, was associated in two probable cases and one possible case in Inman's (1977) report. Reversible cases of purpura, thrombocytopenia, agranulocytosis and pancytopenia have been reported with fenoprofen, and granulocytopenia with fenbufen, and Inman (1977) noted one probable case with ketoprofen. Aplastic anemia has been reported occasionally with fenoprofen (Ashraf et al., 1982). In relation to their extensive usage propionic acids must be regarded as extremely safe in respect to blood dyscrasias.

Aspirin, Fenamates and Mefenamic Acid

Aspirin rarely causes a reversible thrombocytopenia. Fenamates are occasionally associated with thrombocytopenia and autoimmune leukopenia and autoimmune hemolytic anemia has been reported following prolonged treatment with mefenamic acid.

Diclofenac Sodium and Fenclofenac

About 20 hematological reactions to diclofenac sodium were reported by Ciucci (1979) at a time when it was estimated that 10 million patients had been treated with diclofenac. The majority had other associated factors including 5 who were taking a more likely causative drug. Two had non-hematological disease and of 3 with hemolytic anemia 2 had pre-existing disease. Two patients with aplastic anemia died, but one developed symptoms 5 months after the cessation of treatment and had taken many drugs, including a pyrazolone in the interim. Blood dyscrasias have not been associated with fenclofenac.

Piroxicam

In a review Pitts (1979) makes no mention of blood dyscrasias. One instance of aplastic anemia associated with piroxicam was reported by Lee et al. (1982), although a direct relationship was not proved. We have observed severe hemolytic anemia in one patient on concurrent medication with piroxicam and intramuscular gold injections.

Central Nervous System Side Effects

These are among the most common unwanted symptoms associated with indomethacin therapy and include headache, vertigo, somnolence and depression, reversible on withdrawal of treatment (see chapter 4). Much less common (less than 1%) but much more unpleasant are symptoms of psychic disturbance and depersonalisation, which can be very distressing for the patient. Tinnitus is not uncommon and there are reports of hearing and ocular problems.

Central nervous system side effects result from salicylism but rarely occur when salicylate plasma levels are below 20mg/100ml. The first symptom is usually tinnitus; later deafness may occur. If high levels are maintained, headaches, nausea and vomiting, mental confusion and hyperventilation may set in. In cases of prolonged therapy auditory damage may be permanent, especially in elderly patients. Reversible toxic amblyopia has been associated with ibuprofen but a direct relationship has not been proved.

Minor central nervous system side effects do occur with other NSAIDs but these are trivial. It is important to ask about central nervous system side effects early in treatment, especially with indomethacin, because patients do not usually associate this type of effect with their treatment and so may suffer prolonged discomfort quite unnecessarily.

Idiosyncratic Reactions

Aspirin allergy is of 3 types: bronchial asthma, urticaria and angioneurotic edema, and anaphylactic shock. It is particularly likely to occur in patients who have non-drug-induced allergies. Although other NSAIDs will provoke these reactions they are far more likely to occur in patients already sensitive to aspirin (see also chapter 4). It has been postulated that the asthma and urticaria/edema reactions are due to inhibition of prostaglandin E. These substances are not only bronchodilators but also stabilise histamine in mast cells. It is thus not surprising that sensitive subjects react and that there is cross-reactivity between NSAIDs. These reactions rarely occur if NSAIDs are avoided in aspirin-sensitive patients. In these cases the fenamate drugs, which inhibit PGF_2 bronchoconstriction, may be tried although even these have occasionally induced asthma and anaphylaxis.

Severe Skin Reactions

Severe skin reactions include Stevens-Johnson syndrome, erythema multiforme, toxic epidermal necrolysis (Lyell's syndrome) and exfoliative dermatitis.

Weber (1984), using the technique already described, studied reports only for erythema multiforme and toxic epidermal necrolysis. He found them not so rare with fenclofenac and feprazone, with one report for 28,000 to 67,000 prescriptions, less frequent with benoxaprofen and diflunisal (one per 122,000 to 131,000 prescriptions) and very rare or not reported with the remainder.

All these conditions have been reported in association with phenylbutazone therapy. They usually occur within 2 or 3 weeks of the onset of treatment and were reported much more frequently when high dosage was still being used. They are now rare.

Indomethacin has been associated with exfoliative dermatitis, but these severe reactions do not appear to have been reported in association with propionic acids or fenamates. With aspirin, urticaria is common. As with many other NSAIDs mild skin reactions occur in 1 to 2% of patients treated (see also chapter 4) but severe reactions are not a problem. Fenclofenac induces a rash in about 19% of patients and although a proportion can restart treatment without a recurrence, it is the cause for withdrawal in 10% of the patients treated (Swain et al., 1979). Erythema multiforme has been reported and very rarely Stevens-Johnson syndrome and toxic epidermal necrolysis have occurred. The drug has been withdrawn from the market in the United Kingdom because of its propensity to cause skin reactions. Diclofenac sodium very rarely causes skin problems but Ciucci (1979) noted that a fatal case of Stevens-Johnson syndrome had occurred. With piroxicam, some 3% of patients treated develop a rash or pruritus and Stevens-Johnson syndrome has also been reported. In a recent review of cutaneous reactions to NSAIDs reported to the Adverse Drug Reaction Reporting System instituted by the American Academy of Dermatology, Stern and Bigby (1984) analysed 135 reports received between December 1980 and July 1983. There were 2 fatalities, both in patients who developed toxic epidermal necrolysis, one in association with zomepirac and the other with sulindac.

Hepatic Toxicity

Although drug-induced hepatitis is one of the more common causes of jaundice, NSAIDs are among the less frequent offenders. Both cholangitic and hepatitic types have been reported following NSAID therapy. In his report, Weber (1984) used only the term liver damage, not specifying whether this included a simple liver function test abnormality or much more severe derangement. The order of ranking was not dissimilar to that for blood dyscrasias, with feprazone ranked first, and sulindac, benoxaprofen and fenclofenac second (table 3.4).

In a review of 41 cases of phenylbutazone-induced hepatitis (Fowler et al., 1975) there was a predominance of females aged over 50 years. Many cases, particularly the hepatocellular form, had occurred when high dose phenylbutazone was still common. This was not infrequently associated with a generalized sensitivity reaction and carried a very high mortality rate. The cholestatic form usually resolves rapidly when the drug is withdrawn.

A number of cases of toxic hepatitis, some fatal, have been reported with indomethacin. Toxic hepatitis has not been reported with azapropazone or the fenamates and is extremely unusual with propionic acids, although cholestatic jaundice was one of the reasons for the withdrawal of benoxaprofen from the market. High doses of aspirin, especially in children, may lead to an acute but mild reversible hepatocellular injury (Zimmerman, 1974). A small number of cases of jaundice have been reported with diclofenac sodium but all have resolved. During the course of treatment of rheumatoid arthritis with NSAIDs, minor elevations of liver enzymes are a common finding. Alkaline phosphatase, however, behaves like an acute phase protein, and is usually increased in the active phase of the disease, regardless of therapy, to between 100 and 160 iu/L, returning to the normal range as disease activity is controlled. Furthermore, in some cases of very severe rheumatoid arthritis, the liver may (though rarely) be involved in the rheumatoid process when very high enzyme levels may be found.

Table 3.4. The frequency of liver damage (not defined) caused by various NSAIDs: ranked comparisons (Weber, 1984)

Drug	Rank	Approximate no. of prescriptions for one ADR report
Feprazone	1	11,300
Sulindac	2	
Benoxaprofen	2	34,000-69,000
Fenclofenac	2	
Flurbiprofen	3	
Diclofenac	3	110,000-218,000
Azapropazone	3	
Diflunisal	3	
Piroxicam	4	760,000

Renal Toxicity

The kidney is an active site for synthesis and metabolism of prostaglandins which participate in the regulation of renal blood flow, glomerular filtration, renin release, tubular ion transport and water metabolism. Prostaglandins are particularly important when volume contraction caused by salt depletion is present, maintaining renal blood flow and glomerular filtration, as in congestive cardiac failure and cirrhosis with ascites. Reduction of prostaglandin synthesis by NSAIDs has been shown to have little effect on renal function in healthy volunteers with both aspirin and indomethacin, but renal failure has been precipitated in a patient with congestive heart failure treated with indomethacin, as well as in cirrhotic conditions. Non-oliguric renal failure has been observed in elderly patients receiving fenamates who were dehydrated as a result of diarrhea. In nephrotic states plasma volume may be reduced and indomethacin may reduce renal blood flow and glomerular filtration in these patients.

In chronic renal parenchymal disease, active prostaglandin production maximises glomerular filtration. In lupus nephritis, aspirin may reduce creatinine clearance by as much as 58%. Ibuprofen, naproxen and fenoprofen have a similar effect and histological studies have shown acute tubular necrosis superimposed on the glomerular disease. Phenylbutazone has produced acute tubular damage and necrosis both because of its uricosuric effect, with uric acid crystallisation in the tubules and as part of a generalized idiosyncratic reaction.

Renal Papillary Necrosis

Although a number of reports have associated NSAIDs (ibuprofen, indomethacin, phenylbutazone, fenoprofen and mefenamic acid) with this condition, a clear cause and effect relationship has not been established.

NSAID-induced nephrotic syndrome is usually reversible but may require dialysis. Interstitial lymphocytic infiltration, tubular degeneration and minimal glomerular change characterize the condition. It has been reported with fenoprofen, indomethacin, naproxen and tolmetin (Brezin et al., 1979; Cartwright et al., 1979). Nephrotic syndrome was reported in association with fenclofenac with recovery on withdrawal (Smith, 1977) and at least one other similar case has been described.

Reversible elevations of blood urea are common with most NSAIDs and have been studied, for example, with ibuprofen, mefenamic acid and piroxicam. Indomethacin can occasionally produce hyperkalemia.

Overall Findings

Table 3.5 has been prepared from drug symposia reports, manufacturers' summaries and data sheets currently available and interpreted in the light of experience. It does not agree exactly with data from CSM reports (table 3.2) or with Weber's findings, because different sources or interpretations have been used. It is, however, presented here as a reasonable, practical and quick reference guide. Weber's (1984) method is interesting. In his final table he lists the number of times that each drug has appeared in the highest and lowest frequency group of the 5 types of reaction he studied: gastrointestinal hemorrhage, liver damage, blood dyscrasias, nephropathy and severe bullous skin reaction. This is shown in table 3.6. It should be emphasized that these figures concern only the first 2 years after marketing. Whether these findings will continue in the same ratio remains to be seen, although feprazone, fenclofenac and benoxaprofen have already been subjected to legislative action.

Conclusions

Reporting of fatal and severe adverse drug reactions is haphazard, unreliable and influenced by emotional and other factors. Spontaneous reporting cannot be relied on as giving anything but the most approximate estimate of the frequency of the rare severe reactions which occur from time to time with most NSAIDs. Some types of reaction, because of the emotional impact they cause (such as aplastic anemia) are very likely to be reported; others also with a potentially fatal outcome (gastric bleeding and perforation) appear to be acceptable risks and hence are less likely to be reported. Media and consumer association publicity and misinterpretation of medical problems exaggerate this bias.

Table 3.5. Summary of the major adverse effects of commonly used NSAIDs

	Major toxic reactions[a]					
	Blood dyscrasias	CNS side effects	Idiosyncratic reactions	Severe skin reactions	Hepatic toxicity	Renal toxicity
Indomethacin	E	E		E	E	
Diclofenac sodium	I	r		r	I	
Naproxen	I	r		r		R
Piroxicam	I	r		R		r
Ibuprofen	I	I		r		r
Flurbiprofen	N	r		r		
Fenclofenac[b]		r		R		I
Aspirin and variants	I	E	E	r	E	
Phenylbutazone[c] Oxyphenbutazone[b]	E	r		E	E	
Azapropazone	N	r		r	N	
Fenamates		r	0	r	N	
Feprazone[b]	E			r		
Fenoprofen	R/E	r		r		R
Fenbufen	R	r		r		
Ketoprofen	I	r		r		r

a *Key to symbols:* 0 = do not occur; r = reported but minor; E = established; R = reported; N = not reported; I = isolated reports; Blank = no data.
b Withdrawn from the market in the UK.
c Withdrawn except for treatment of ankylosing spondylitis in hospitalized patients.

It is, of course, virtually impossible to prove negative associations. Large clinical trials without serious incidents at many centers may purport to show the safety of a particular drug, but these are unlikely to identify events occurring once in, say, 72,000 patient-years of treatment. Medications that have been used extensively for many years are thus likely to have many more associated reports than recent introductions.

Clearly, it is possible to establish certain degrees of risk, and acceptable risks are certainly related to efficacy however difficult these are to define. But this is not the only criterion. A relatively high risk, say one death per 100,000 treatments, does not become a hazard if the drug is not extensively used. But, as we have seen with phenylbutazone, this frequency for a high

Table 3.6. Number of times specific NSAIDs have appeared in the most or least frequently reported adverse reaction group (Weber, 1984)

Drug	Most frequently reported group	Least frequently reported group
Feprazone	5	0
Fenclofenac	4	0
Benoxaprofen	3	0
Azapropazone	2	2
Diflunisal	1	0
Flurbiprofen	1	2
Piroxicam	1	3
Diclofenac	0	2
Sulindac	0	1

rate prescription item may result in, say, 20 deaths per annum, and over a period of years becomes unacceptable, even for a most efficacious preparation.

Where potentially fatal reactions are concerned we have to accept the real risk of blood dyscrasias with pyrazole drugs, therefore they should be reserved only for very special indications and specific patients. Indomethacin is probably still the most effective NSAID, but does have the potential for severe gastrointestinal toxicity, though much of this can be minimized by careful selection and supervision of patients. The older established propionic acids naproxen and ibuprofen have stood up well to the test of time and two of the rather newer preparations, diclofenac sodium and piroxicam, also appear to be establishing a good effect : safety ratio.

References

Adams, S.S. and Warwick-Buckler, J.: Ibuprofen and flurbiprofen; in Huskisson (Ed.) Anti-Rheumatic Drugs (Praeger, New York 1983).

Ashraf, M.; Pearson, R.M. and Winfield, D.A.: Aplastic anaemia associated with fenoprofen. British Medical Journal 284: 1301-1302 (1982).

Babb, J.; Bishop, H.; Schneider, R.E.; Hawkins, C.F. and Hoare, A.M.: Plasma propranolol levels in inflammatory disease. Lancet 1: 1413 (1976).

Brezin, J.H.; Katz, S.M.; Schwartz, A.B. and Chinitz, J.L.: Reversible renal failure and nephrotic syndrome associated with non-steroidal anti-inflammatory drugs. New England Journal of Medicine 301: 1271-1273 (1979).

Cartwright, K.C.; Trotter, T.L. and Cohen, M.L.: Naproxen nephrotoxicity. Arizona Medicine 36: 124-126 (1979).

Ciucci, A.: A review of spontaneously reported adverse drug reactions. Rheumatology and Rehabilitation (Suppl. 2): 116-121 (1979).

Committee on Safety of Medicines: Personal communication (1984).
Fowler, P.D.: Marrow toxicity of the pyrazoles. Annals of the Rheumatic Diseases 26: 344 (1967).
Fowler, P.D. and Faragher, E.B.: Drug and non-drug factors influencing adverse reactions to pyrazoles. Journal of International Medical Research 5 (Suppl. 2): 108-120 (1977).
Fowler, P.D.; Woolfe, D. and Alexander, S.: Phenylbutazone and hepatitis. Rheumatology and Rehabilitation 14: 71-75 (1975).
Girdwood, R.H.: Death after taking medicaments. British Medical Journal 1: 501-504 (1974).
Inman, W.H.I.: Study of fatal bone-marrow depression with special reference to phenylbutazone and oxyphenbutazone. British Medical Journal 1: 1500-1507 (1977).
Lee, S.H.; Fawcett, V. and Preese, J.M.: Aplastic anaemia associated with piroxicam. Lancet 1: 1186 (1982).
Mason, R.M.: The treatment of gout. Prescriber's Journal 7: 125-131 (1968).
Pitts, N.E.: Review of clinical trial experiences with piroxicam; in Symposium Proceedings IXth European Congress of Rheumatology Wiesbaden, p.48 (Academy Professional Information Services 1979).
Smith, R.B.: Analysis of side effect patterns presenting during the course of a continuing long term open study of fenclofenac. Proceedings of the Royal Society of Medicine 70 (Suppl. 6): 46-48 (1977).
Stern, R.S. and Bigby, M.: Cutaneous reactions to non-steroidal anti-inflammatory drugs. Journal of the American Medical Association 252: 1433-1437 (1984).
Swain, M.C.; Goldberg, A.A.J. and Smith, D.W.: Fenclofenac: A 5 year review of patient tolerance; in Fenclofenac: International Congress and Symposium Series No.28, p.73 (Royal Society of Medicine, Academic Press 1979).
Weber, J.C.P.: Epidemiology of adverse reactions to non-steroidal anti-inflammatory drugs; in Rainsford and Velo (Eds) Advances in Inflammation Research, vol. 6 (Raven Press, New York 1984).
Zimmerman, H.J.: Aspirin induced hepatic injury. Annals of Internal Medicine 80: 103-105 (1974).

4. Incidence of Minor Toxicity

Hedley Berry

King's College Hospital, London, England

It is accepted that drugs cause side effects, but under what circumstances are those side effects acceptable? In potentially fatal situations (e.g. the treatment of pneumonia by penicillin) the risk is acceptable if there are no other agents capable of producing the desired clinical effect without causing side effects. A similar situation is seen with severe rheumatoid arthritis where the only available disease-modifying antirheumatoid agents cause major side effects, but these drugs are considered acceptable and are in current usage.

With the non-steroidal anti-inflammatory drugs (NSAIDs), the situation is different. Often they are prescribed for minor ailments, the odd pain or ache which will in time improve on its own. In that situation it could be argued that a drug causing side effects should not be prescribed. There is a strong argument for being certain that the ratio of cost in terms of side effects to benefit in terms of efficacy is an acceptable one.

Factors Influencing the Perception of Drug Reactions

On the basis of the considerable available information, there is no NSAID which is both effective and free of side effects. However, two important factors influence our perception of the incidence of side effects both in an absolute sense and relative to other NSAIDs.

Dosage

There has been a tendency for NSAIDs to be recommended at subtherapeutic dosage at the time of marketing. An example of this was ibuprofen which was originally marketed at a recommended dose of 200mg three times a day. At this dosage the number of side effects encountered were few; on the other hand its clinical effectiveness was also negligible. Doubling the dose appeared neither to produce more side effects nor much more in the way of clinical efficacy. For a long time this remained the prescribed dose of the drug in general practice. It might be argued that the response sought was a placebo response and that the pink pills produced this placebo response which was useful to the patients. More recently, trials of this drug at 1600mg per day in the author's hands have confirmed that it is still only equal to placebo, and only at 2.4g per day does the drug begin to have proper effectiveness, as judged by anti-inflammatory activity. At this dose side effects encountered are similar to those seen with other NSAIDs.

Similarly, naproxen was originally used at a dosage of 250mg twice daily but now the recommended dose is 500mg two or three times daily. Likewise with indomethacin which was often prescribed at a dosage of 25mg twice daily and now is sometimes administered as 50mg three times a day. Unfortunately, the literature is bedevilled with trials at dosages that have been subtherapeutic, particularly of comparative agents (see chapter 2). It is impossible, therefore, to derive much useful data about the true incidence of side effects from such studies. Not all NSAIDs at the time of marketing have been subjected to the rigorous clinical trials that one would have expected (chapter 2). Necessarily, these include dose ranging studies against placebo, comparative drug studies also involving placebo (preferably using the double-blind crossover or parallel group technique). The 'numbers game' is also important here to make sure that sufficient patients are recruited to avoid a type 2 error. Finally, a large tolerance study over a fixed time period with known dosage to assess side effects should be carried out, probably in general practice to reproduce the more 'everyday' conditions of use.

Public Reaction

There is commercial risk in marketing a drug at an acceptable dosage where efficacy is the major concern. The number of side effects produced may mean that the drug becomes 'unacceptable'. Who is to decide this degree of acceptability? There has been a tendency in recent times for the media, at least in the United Kingdom, to have an unacceptably strong influence. It should be the Committee on Safety of Medicines and the Committee of Review of Medicines that make the decision independent of such outside pressures.

We have recently seen the withdrawal of some highly effective compounds. Phenylbutazone and oxyphenbutazone were withdrawn from general use because they caused aplastic anemia (see table 1.1; p.11). There had been reports of at least 500 deaths associated with phenylbutazone in the United Kingdom alone since it was introduced in 1952 (see also chapter 3). Indoprofen caused an unacceptably high incidence of gastrointestinal irritation with peptic ulceration, hematemesis and melena. Perhaps the most outstanding example of the media pressure was the demise of benoxaprofen. This drug, seemingly having both cyclo-oxygenase- and lipoxygenase-inhibiting properties, was withdrawn in a blaze of negative publicity partly relating to the very rare incidence of the hepatorenal syndrome, partly due to its ability to cause perforation and gastrointestinal intolerance (no more than many other NSAIDs), and partly because of its effect on the elderly, in whom the drug was found to be present in the blood in higher levels, persisting for longer periods than in the younger population. The main problem was blanket exposure as a result of the original launch leading to half a million patients receiving the drug very rapidly. This may be the best way of carrying out a toxicity study or marketing surveillance study, but it does expose drugs to major risks. Fenclofenac and feprazone have also been withdrawn in the United Kingdom. One wonders whether aspirin if released now and submitted to the Committee on Safety of Medicines would have ever been granted a clinical trial certificate, let alone a product licence.

Gastrointestinal Side Effects

The gastroscope has been helpful in the evaluation of the comparative gastrointestinal toxicity risk. Studies have been carried out using regular aspirin as well as the newer and special forms (e.g. enteric-coated preparations or buffered, glycinated or micro-crystalline forms). Regular aspirin is the most likely of all NSAIDs to produce areas of irritative and superficial erosion in the stomach (Lanza et al., 1980).

Comparing the gastroscopic effects of naproxen, indomethacin, aspirin and ibuprofen after one week of medication in 40 normal volunteers, aspirin, 3.6g per day, was found to be the worst in terms of its ability to cause gastric mucosal damage (Lanza et al., 1979b) [fig. 4.1]. A further study by the same author found considerable gastric erosive change with tolmetin in 2 out of 5 subjects, the other 3 patients showing less extensive but definite change.

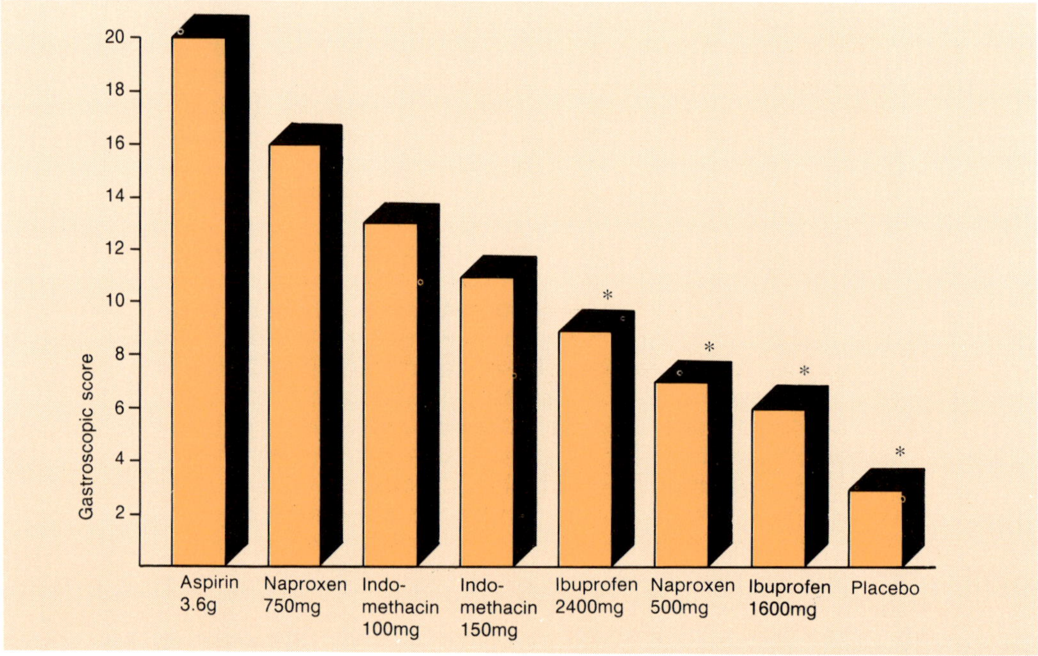

Fig 4.1. Relative gastroscopic score (according to degree of gastric mucosal damage) after 1 week's administration of aspirin 3.6 g/day, naproxen 500 and 750 mg/day, indomethacin 100 and 150 mg/day, ibuprofen 1600 and 2400 mg/day or placebo to 40 healthy subjects studied under single-blind conditions. Asterisks indicate a significantly lesser effect than aspirin (data from Lanza et al., 1979b).

Ibuprofen was better tolerated, showing erosive gastritis in only 1 patient, the other 4 having minimal and mild changes. It was noted that the symptoms correlated poorly with gastroscopic findings (Lanza et al., 1979a).

Gastroscopic findings in normal, rheumatoid arthritic and osteoarthritic patients are similar in that aspirin appears to be the most irritant of all the NSAIDs. The route of administration may also influence the incidence of gastric effects; indomethacin suppositories, for example, cause no more gastric irritation than placebo but the capsules cause significantly more (Lanza et al., 1982) [see chapter 5]. There is, however, some dispute as to whether indomethacin serum concentrations are lower after administration of the suppository than of the capsule.

It is often difficult to assess the true incidence of nausea, dyspepsia, epigastric pain or for that matter gastric ulceration and bleeding from the published data. Some 13% of more than 73,000 patients who were receiving piroxicam in post-marketing surveillance studies exhibited one or other of these problems (Brogden et al., 1984). It is extremely hard to determine the incidence of peptic ulceration in view of variable dosage regimens and length of exposure to drugs. Other concurrent drug therapy needs to be taken into account and a comparison made with patients developing ulcers who are not taking NSAIDs. It is unclear whether rheumatoid arthritis itself renders patients more likely to develop peptic ulceration. 'Silent' ulcers have been encountered in gastroscopy studies in the author's unit. Even so, there is a suggestion that the overall incidence of peptic ulceration and gastrointestinal hemorrhage in patients with chronic rheumatic disease on NSAIDs appears to be somewhere between 0.1 and 0.2% (Ando et al., 1983). This has been looked at particularly carefully with piroxicam. In patients receiving higher dosages than 20mg daily (the recommended normal dose), the incidence went up to 7% (Pisko et al., 1980). A careful study using the medicines division of the Department of Health data (Weber, 1984) has been carried out (see chapter 3). Gastrointestinal hemorrhage or perforation appears to occur in one in 9500 to 17,000 prescriptions. Patients receiving piroxicam, feprazone, azapropazone, diflunisal, fenclofenac and flurbiprofen were studied (see also chapter 3, tables 3.3, 3.4 and 3.6). With piroxicam, upper gastrointestinal bleeding has been seen more commonly in elderly patients than younger patients on 20mg daily (Emery and Grahame, 1982; Laakae et al., 1984; Ward and Weir, 1982). It seems reasonable to suggest that caution should be employed when prescribing NSAIDs in the elderly.

Constipation and Diarrhea

The incidence of lower bowel problems in patients treated with NSAIDs is also hard to define. There is a suggestion, for example, that indomethacin may cause diarrhea in some patients. This is also encountered on occasion with ketoprofen, naproxen, fenclofenac, feprazone, flufenamic acid, mefenamic acid, flurbiprofen, sulindac and tiaprofenic acid. What interpretation to put on this is not known as whether patients are more inclined to report diarrhea than constipation is hard to assess.

Dermatological Problems

Nonspecific skin eruptions are frequently seen in patients treated with NSAIDs. Other dermatological side effects include pruritus, phototoxicity and erythema multiforme, as well as the more rare serious reactions discussed in chapter 3. Angioedema as well as urticaria has been reported in patients on aspirin. The rash seen with indomethacin varies from an erythema to one which is maculopapular; urticaria has also been reported. Phenylbutazone has been associated with urticaria as well as severe skin reactions. Naproxen has been reported as causing angioedema and even rarely alopecia, along with facial edema and urticaria. Piroxicam has been linked to photosensitivity reactions, erythematous rashes and also angioedema and alopecia. There have also been numerous reports of urticaria. Ibuprofen has also been reported as causing angioedema, urticaria and rash. Azapropazone has most commonly been associated with photosensitivity reactions and erythematous and maculopapular rashes; occasional urticaria is also reported. Diclofenac has been associated with maculopapular rashes and urticaria, as has diflunisal. Fenclofenac has been frequently associated with maculopapular rashes and urticaria, as has feprazone. It is difficult to obtain an overall incidence of dermatological side effects, but a figure of 0.8% is quoted from various large multicentre studies.

Skin Reactions with Benoxaprofen

Certain NSAIDs, namely alclofenac, fenclofenac and benoxaprofen (which was also associated with other effects, see below), have been withdrawn because of a high incidence of skin reactions. Benoxaprofen provoked photosensitivity reactions particularly in fair-skinned people. Halsey and Cardoe (1982) reported that cutaneous side effects occurred frequently in their series of 300 patients and accounted for 180 of all the 259 side effects they reported. Photosensitivity occurred in 86 patients. Toxic side effects were in general more common in the elderly (fig. 4.2). Photosensitivity, however, occurred more often in patients under 70 years of age though this may have been due to less exposure to sun in the older group. Onycholysis, koilonychia and milia were all reported with benoxaprofen. Of the 180 cutaneous side effects reported in this series in all age groups, 47% were due to photosensitivity, 14.4% to rashes and 8.8% to milia (multi subepidermal cysts). Less commonly reported were koilonychia, increased hair and nail growth, pruritus, erythema multiforme, Stevens-Johnson syndrome and toxic epidermal necrolysis.

In the elderly there were more gastrointestinal than cutaneous toxic reactions and there were several fatal cases of cholestatic jaundice, which was a major reason for its withdrawal.

Of interest was that severe extensive psoriasis resistant to all therapy improved in 7 of 14 patients on this agent. Seven failed to improve of whom one developed erythema multiforme. In the patients who did respond it was rapid and dramatic. Five of the original 14 were cleared of otherwise intractable psoriasis.

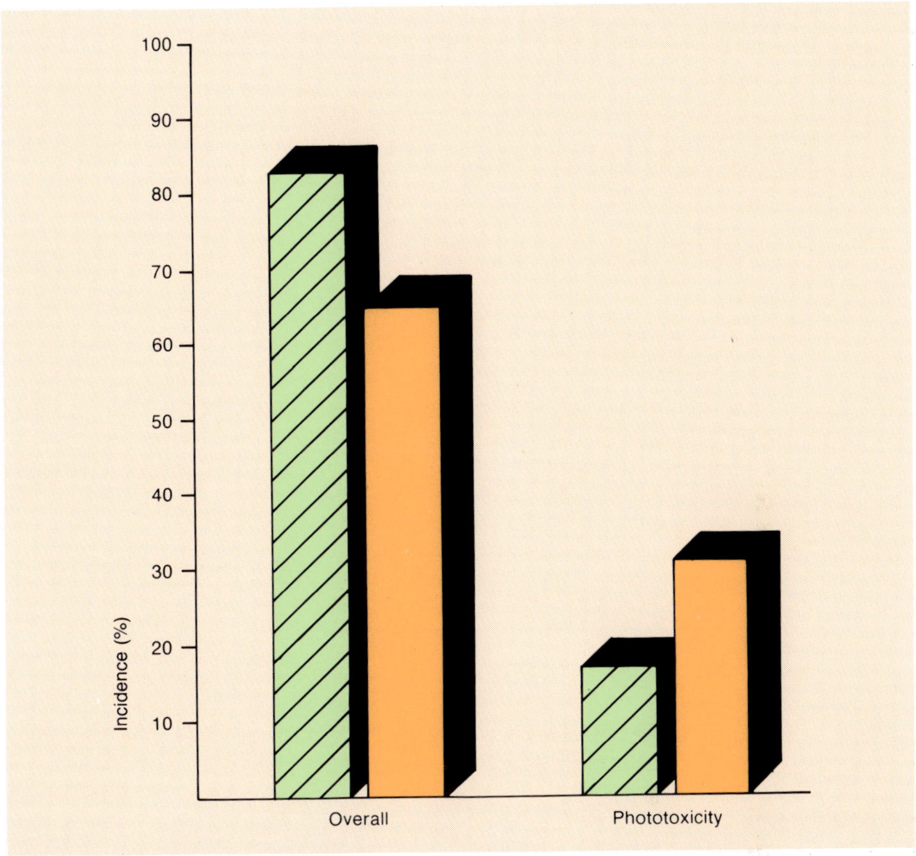

Fig. 4.2 Relative incidence of all side effects and of phototoxicity among 42 elderly patients (>70 years) ▨ and 258 younger patients (< 70 years) ☐ treated with benoxaprofen (data from Halsley and Cardoe, 1982).

Other Side Effects

Renal side effects thought to be associated with non-steroidal anti-inflammatory drugs in patients with normal renal function are rare. However, a wide range of clinical renal syndromes may occasionally be associated with the use of the NSAIDs, particularly in patients with pre-existing renal disease. These are discussed in chapter 3. Caution should be exercised in prescribing NSAIDs to patients at risk of developing renal complications, such as those with chronic renal insufficiency, congestive heart failure, hepatic cirrhosis, and volume contraction secondary to the nephrotic syndrome or diuretic use. Recent studies in patients with chronic glomerular nephritis and mild renal insufficiency demonstrated that sulindac produced no fall in glomerular filtration rate or renal blood flow, and it is possible that this drug may offer an advantage in this area over other NSAIDs (Ciabattoni et al., 1984).

Exacerbation of Asthma

The complication of bronchoconstriction, occurring particularly in asthmatic patients with aspirin hypersensitivity, has been described most recently with zomepirac and has led to the withdrawal of this drug (see chapter 1; table 1.1). It has rarely been seen, however, with other NSAIDs.

Drug Interactions

Anticoagulants

Few serious drug interactions have been described with non-steroidal anti-inflammatory drugs. However, one area where there have been many reports is where NSAIDs have been added to regimens of patients already receiving anticoagulant therapy (table 4.1). One particular early study involv-

Table 4.1. Clinically important interactions with NSAIDs (adapted from Hart, 1980)

Drug	May interact with	Potential result
Oral anticoagulants	Aspirin	Salicylates have no clinically important effect on anticoagulant control, but should be avoided because they increase risk of bleeding by affecting platelet function.
	Phenylbutazone Oxyphenbutazone	Predictable and significant prolongation of prothrombin time of coumarins and risk of hemorrhage
Oral sulfonylurea hypoglycemic agents	Aspirin	Activity of sulfonylurea may be increased with ***large doses*** of aspirin
Phenytoin	Phenylbutazone Oxyphenbutazone	Probably a predictable increase in hypoglycemic activity
	Phenylbutazone Oxyphenbutazone Azapropazone	In a few cases, there may be a marked increase in plasma phenytoin concentrations
Adrenergic neurone blocking antihypertensive drugs (e.g. guanethidine)	Phenylbutazone Oxyphenbutazone	Antihypertensive effect may be antagonized (fluid retention) and control of blood pressure may be lost
Antacids	Aspirin	Absorbable and non-absorbable antacids, markedly increase urinary excretion of salicylate so that therapeutic serum levels can not be maintained
Probenecid	Indomethacin	Increases plasma concentrations of indomethacin and enhances pain relief without increasing or less CNS effects
Corticosteroids	Aspirin	Decreased plasma salicylate levels due to more rapid rate of salicylate metabolism; accumulation of salicylate with risk of toxicity when corticosteroid dosage decreased and salicylate dosage not modified
Probenecid	Salicylates (low doses)	Therapeutic efficacy of uricosuric agent markedly inhibited

ing such combination therapy (Holmes, 1966) shows that patients who received mefenamic acid or aspirin had increased bleeding and clotting times as a result of these drugs. Similar reports have appeared for many NSAIDs particularly phenylbutazone and oxyphenbutazone. Based on current evidence, the safest NSAIDs in anticoagulated patients are probably ibuprofen, naproxen and tolmetin. In doses of 800 to 1200mg daily tolmetin does not appear to affect the hypoprothrombinemic response to oral anticoagulants (Ascione, 1978; Pullar and Capell, 1983). Naproxen administration was not associated with changes in the pharmacokinetics or hypoprothrombinemic response to warfarin in 10 healthy subjects treated with warfarin for 25 days and who received naproxen 375mg bid from day 11 to day 20 (Jain et al., 1979). In another study, naproxen (375mg bid for 17 days) failed to affect the pharmacokinetics or anticoagulant effect of a single 5mg dose of warfarin (Slattery et al., 1979). Similarly, ibuprofen may not affect the hypoprothrombinemic response to oral anticoagulants and is probably one of the safer NSAIDs to use (Boekhout-Mussert and Loeliger, 1974). However, the potentially adverse effects of these drugs on the gastric mucosa (see above) and platelet function in the anticoagulated patient should be considered.

Drugs for which there is some clinical evidence of an increase in the hypoprothrombinemic response to anticoagulants but for which the incidence and/or magnitude is not known include meclofenamate, sulindac, diflunisal, piroxicam and mefenamic acid.

It is thus reasonable to suggest that any patient who receives an NSAID whilst receiving anticoagulant therapy should be very carefully monitored, as all NSAIDs inhibit platelet function.

Digitalis

Digitalis glycosides have also been studied in some detail. There is evidence that indomethacin has induced digitalis toxicity possibly by impairment of renal function by indomethacin (Schimmol et al., 1980). Further work showed a marked reduction in serum digitoxin levels caused by the concurrent use of phenylbutazone.

Hypoglycemics

Although aspirin can cause lower blood glucose levels, small analgesic doses have not been reported to cause excessive hypoglycemia. Some modification of the hypoglycemic agent dosage might be necessary if large doses are used, but reports of adverse interactions with aspirin in therapeutic doses appear to be lacking. Prolonged hypoglycemic coma has been reported when phenylbutazone is administered with sulfonylureas, probably due to inhibition of metabolism of the sulfonylurea (Ober, 1974). Oxyphenbutazone and azapropazone (Andreasen et al., 1981) apparently have a similar effect on tolbutamide metabolism.

Antacids and Laxatives

Antacids and laxatives have also been looked at; dihydroxyaluminum sodium carbonate, magnesium-aluminum silicate, bisacodyl and anthraquinone laxatives do not interact significantly with azapropazone.

However, concurrent administration of aspirin and calcium and magnesium hydroxide, calcium carbonate or sodium bicarbonate may decrease plasma salicylate concentrations in patients with rheumatoid arthritis or rheumatic fever through increases in urinary pH (see chapter 5). The systemic bioavailability of diflunisal is decreased by concomitant administration of aluminum hydroxide and absorption of naproxen is decreased by concurrent magnesium oxide or aluminum hydroxide, but not by a magnesium-aluminum hydroxide gel.

NSAIDs and Aspirin

Is there any problem of interaction between NSAIDs and aspirin? Coadministration of aspirin with other NSAIDs has been reported to decrease the plasma concentrations of diflunisal, naproxen, fenoprofen, ketoprofen, fenbufen, flurbiprofen, ibuprofen, diclofenac and mefenamic acid, although the clinical significance of these findings is uncertain. The uricosuric effects of phenylbutazone and aspirin are mutually antagonized by concurrent use. Aspirin may also diminish the uricosuric action of probenecid and sulfinpyrazone.

Frequency of Side Effects in Relation to Total Drug Exposure

Compared with aspirin, other NSAIDs have a lower incidence of side effects although there is a tendency for phenylbutazone, oxyphenbutazone and indomethacin to have more than others (see chapter 3). For example, comparing total side effects with indomethacin and piroxicam gave an incidence of 15% with piroxicam and 22% with indomethacin (Brogden et at., 1984) and in long term studies with diclofenac and indomethacin, treatment was withdrawn because of adverse effects in 6.5% of diclofenac patients and 13% of indomethacin patients (Brogden et al., 1980). Analysis of controlled therapeutic trials comparing the newer NSAIDs suggests that all these drugs cause a similar incidence of side effects. As a subgroup the propionic acids seem especially well tolerated – but this generalization must be re-examined in the light of the benoxaprofen experience.

The question of the extent to which side effects are dose-related is important. Figure 4.3 shows such a relationship for the gastrointestinal side effects of piroxicam. By contrast, the side effects of naproxen appear not to be dose-related (Hazleman et al., 1979; Luftschein et al., 1979; Mowat et al., 1984).

Future pharmaceutical development may produce compounds with less toxic potential. Several agents under investigation are claimed to be safer

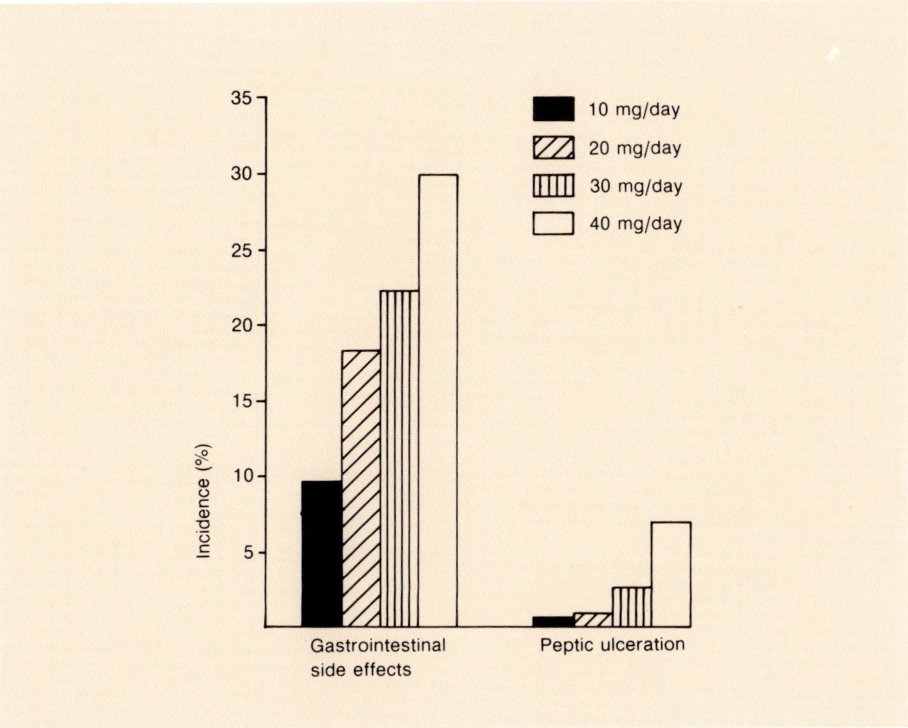

Fig. 4.3 Incidence of gastrointestinal side effects and peptic ulcer relative to piroxicam dosage in patients with rheumatic diseases (Brogden et al., 1984).

than the established drugs and it will be interesting to see whether the initial promise of etodolac, a structurally novel NSAID, which has been reported to produce significantly less gastrointestinal bleeding than indomethacin, naproxen or ibuprofen (Arnold et al., 1983) is fulfilled in clinical practice.

There is an old English proverb – 'You get naught for naught'. This would appear to be valid in the use of all drugs, particularly the NSAIDs. The view of this writer is that NSAIDs cause a large number of minor side effects but generally few severe side effects. Each prescription must be based on a valid judgement that the therapeutic indication outweighs the possible risk of side effects.

References

Ando, G.; Jellheden, B. and Sodergren, J.: Toleration of piroxicam. International Medicine 3: 37-41 (1983).

Andreasen, P.B.; Simonsen, K.; Brocks, K.; Dimo, B. and Bouchelouche, P.: Hypoglycaemia induced by azapropazone-tolbutamide interaction. British Journal of Clinical Pharmacology 12: 581-583 (1981)

Arnold, J.; Weidler, D.; Mullane, J.; Meinders, J.; Jallad, N.; Gard, D.; Hayden, D.; Perdamo, C.; Rumo, T. and Burger, A.: Comparison of etodolac, ibuprofen, indomethacin and naproxen on intestinal microbleeding in normal males. Clinical Pharmacology and Therapeutics 33: 266 (1983).

Ascione, F.J.: Oral anticoagulants with aspirin alternatives. Drug Therapy 8 (No. 9): 152-157 (1978).

Boekhout-Mussert, M.J. and Loeliger, E.A.: Influence of ibuprofen on oral anti-coagulation with phenprocoumon. Journal of International Medical Research 2: 279-283 (1974).

Brogden, R.N.; Heel, R.C.; Pakes, G.E.; Speight, T.M. and Avery G.S.: Diclofenac sodium: A review. Drugs 20: 24-48 (1980).

Brogden, R.N.; Heel, R.C.; Speight, T.M. and Avery, G.S.: Piroxicam – A re-appraisal of its rheumatology and therapeutic efficacy. Drugs 28: 292-323 (1984).

Ciabattoni, G.; Cinotti, G.A.; Pierucci, A.; Simonetti, B.M.; Manzi, M.; Pugliese, F.; Barsotti, P.; Pecci, G.; Taggi, T. and Patrono, C.: Effects of sulindac and ibuprofen in patients with chronic glomerular disease. New England Journal of Medicine 310: 279-283 (1984).

Emery, P. and Grahame, R.: Gastro-intestinal blood loss and piroxicam. Lancet I: 1302-1303 (1982).

Halsey, J.P. and Cadoe, N.: Benoxaprofen – side effects profile in 300 patients. British Medical Journal 284: 1365-1369 (1982).

Hart, F.D.: Rheumatic disorders; in Avery (Ed.) Drug Treatment, 2nd ed., pp.846-888 (ADIS Press, Sydney 1980).

Hazleman, B.L.; Mowat, A.G.; Sturge, R.A.; Hall, M.; Seifert, M.H.; Liyanage, S.P.; Mathews, J.A.; Jenner, J.R. and Engler, C.: A long-term trial of a higher dose of naproxen in the treatment of rheumatoid arthritis, ankylosing spondylitis and osteoarthritis. European Journal of Rheumatology and Inflammation 2: 56-64 (1979).

Holmes, E.I.: Pharmacology of the fenamates. Tolerance by normal human subjects. Annals of Physical Medicine 9 (Suppl): 36 (1966).

Jain, A.; McMahon, G.; Slattery, J.T. and Levy, G.: Effect of naproxen on the steady-state serum concentration and anticoagulant activity of warfarin. Clinical Pharmacology and Therapeutics 25: 61-66 (1979).

Laakae, K.; Kjeldaas, L. and Borchgrevink, C.F.: Side effects of piroxicam. Acta Medica Scandinavica 215: 81-83 (1984).

Lanza, F.L.; Nelson, R.S. and Roger, G.L.: Effect of ibuprofen and placebo on the gastric mucosa of aspirin sensitive volunteers. American Journal of Gastroenterology 72: 528-534 (1979a).

Lanza, F.L.; Roger, G.L.; Nelson, R.S.; Chan, T.T.; Sackman, C. and Rack, M.F.: The effect of ibuprofen, indomethacin, aspirin, naproxen and placebo on the gastric mucosa of normal volunteers. Digestive Diseases and Sciences 24: 823-828 (1979b).

Lanza, F.L.; Roger, G.L. and Nelson, R.S.: Endoscopic evaluation of the side effects of aspirin, buffered aspirin and enteric coated aspirin on gastric and duodenal mucosa. New England Journal of Medicine 303: 136-138 (1980).

Lanza, F.L.; Umben-Haver, E.R.; Nelson, B.B.; Rack, M.F.; Danino, C.P. and White, L.A.: A double-blind randomised placebo controlled gastroscopic study to compare the effects of indomethacin capsules and indomethacin suppositories on the gastric mucosa of human volunteers. Journal of Rheumatology 9: 415-419 (1982).

Luftschein, S.; Bienenstock, H.; Varady, J.C. and Stitt, F.W.: Increasing dose of naproxen in rheumatoid arthritis: Use with and without corticosteroids. Journal of Rheumatology 6: 397-404 (1979).

Mowat, A.M.; Mowat, A.G.; Jones, C.W. and Engler, C.: A comparison of once and twice daily naproxen in rheumatoid arthritis. British Journal of Clinical Practice 38: 95-98 (1984).

Ober, K.F.: Mechanism of interaction of tolbutamide and phenylbutazone in diabetic patients. European Journal of Clinical Pharmacology 7: 291-296 (1974).

Pisko, E.J.; Rahman, M.A.; Turner, R.A. and Agudelo, C.A.: Long term efficacy and safety of piroxicam in the treatment of rheumatoid arthritis. Current Therapeutic Research 27: 852-859 (1980).

Pullar, T. and Capell, H.A.: Interaction between oral anti-coagulant drugs and non-steroidal anti-inflammatory agents: A review. Scottish Medical Journal 28: 42-47 (1983).

Schimmel, M.S.; Inwood, R.J.; Eidelman, A.I. and Fylath, U.: Toxic digitalis levels associated with indomethacin therapy in a neonate. Clinical Pediatrics 19: 768-769 (1980).

Slattery, J.T.; Levy,G.; Jain, A. and McMahon, F.G.: Effect of naproxen on the kinetics of elimination and anticoagulant activity of a single dose of warfarin. Clinical Pharmacology and Therapeutics 25: 51-60 (1979).

Ward, K. and Weir, D.G.: Piroxicam and upper gastro-intestinal haemorrhage. Irish Medical Journal 75: 10-11 (1982).

Weber, J.C.P.: Epidemiology of adverse reactions to non steroidal anti-inflammatory drugs; in Rainsford and Velo (Eds) Advances in Inflammation Research, vol. 6, p.7 (Raven Press, New York 1984).

5. Pharmacokinetic and Chemical Properties of NSAIDs

Peter A. Simkin

Department of Medicine, University of Washington, Seattle, Washington, USA

The ultimate goal of rheumatologic research remains the prevention of each rheumatic disease. While we await this utopian state, rational pharmacologic therapy serves as a formidable but somewhat more realistic intermediate objective. The attainment of such progress can lead to cure (as in septic arthritis) or to control (as in gout) of devastating articular diseases. As in these examples, rational therapy becomes possible when we understand the logic of the underlying disease and the properties of the appropriate therapeutic agent.

At present, however, the causes of most rheumatic diseases are not known. Their pathophysiology yields increasing harvests of relevant findings, but too many barren areas remain. We should not be surprised or discouraged, therefore, by the fact that so many available agents of proven partial effectiveness were first found by chance or during the pursuit of seriously flawed hypotheses. We can expect that therapy will move from empiricism into rationality as and when the underlying logic of rheumatic diseases becomes clear. Until then, we must continue to fight unseen enemies with limited and potentially dangerous weapons.

The drugs reviewed in this publication are aimed not at the cause but at a principal manifestation of rheumatic disease – inflammation. After centuries of study, we still have no better criteria of inflammation than the classical cardinal signs: heat, swelling, redness and pain. It is in these terms that we must evaluate potential anti-inflammatory agents in laboratory animals. It is to control these findings that we administer NSAIDs to patients with rheumatic diseases. Inflammation, however, is not a specific pathologic event but a complex web of participating factors. A host of identified mediators may interact with a multiplicity of potential target cells en route to the microvascular changes we recognize as heat, swelling and erythema. The complexity of these relationships offers a myriad of potential sites where NSAIDs might intervene to reduce the signs of inflammation.

In view of this complexity, it is not surprising that NSAIDs may vary in effectiveness against specific rheumatic diseases or among patients who suffer from the same disease. What is surprising is the fact that a large and seemingly diverse family of pharmacologic agents are so alike in their potential both for desirable anti-inflammatory effects and for unwanted toxic reactions across a broad spectrum of clinical situations. These similarities suggest that the many roads to inflammation converge along limited pathways which offer both shared opportunities for intervention and common risks of serious side effects.

In this chapter we will review some of the pharmacokinetic differences and chemical similarities which may ultimately help us to understand the nature of these pathways and thus the therapeutic and toxic properties of NSAIDs.

Pharmacokinetics

Basic Outline

The pharmacokinetics of individual NSAIDs have been covered in a recent comprehensive review (Verbeeck et al., 1983). The present discussion will focus more on basic principles of this type of work. When appropriate or necessary, specific examples will be cited. Each of these cases is discussed in greater detail by Verbeeck et al. (1983).

Since NSAIDs are generally administered via the alimentary tract (oral tablets or capsules and rectal suppositories), parenteral pharmacokinetics need not be discussed. Most conventional data are derived from curves plotting plasma concentration against time. After oral administration, plasma levels rise to a peak as the agent is absorbed from the intestinal tract. There is then a relatively rapid fall in plasma levels as the drug is distributed through body compartments, and finally a more prolonged decline follows as the agent is metabolized and/or excreted from the body. These 3 phases (absorption, distribution, and elimination) are not distinct in time but overlap significantly with each other (fig 5.1).

Absorption

With rare exceptions, pharmacokinetic studies are begun in the morning and performed in fasting healthy subjects, and less often, patients. In clinical practice however, NSAIDs are often given with or after meals and this factor usually prolongs gastrointestinal uptake. Similarly, antacid administration to dyspeptic individuals may be expected to alter the absorption phase although the available data indicate that such agents are as likely to accelerate as to retard absorption. Unlike some other oral drugs (such as tetracycline), NSAIDs are not bound irretrievably by food and absorption is virtually complete. Clinicians thus need not be concerned that concurrent alimentary intake will deprive the patient of a significant portion of ingested drug. For the most part, fasting enteric absorption is from the stomach and upper small intestine although reliable human data are rarely available and it is likely that the presence of food may alter the site as well as the timing of drug uptake.

Increasingly, NSAIDs are being formulated in sustained-release preparations. Such formulations are designed to circumvent gastric toxicity (see chapters 3 and 4) and to extend the duration of single doses. The goal of

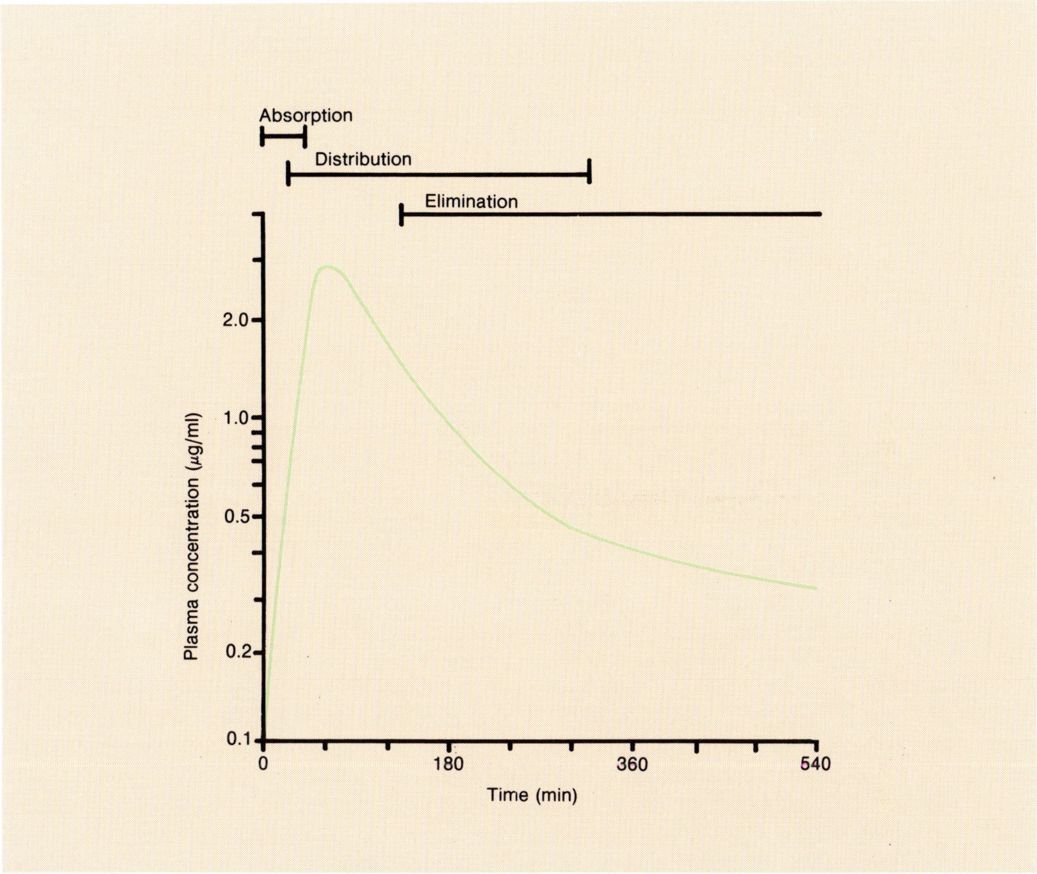

Fig. 5.1. Plasma pharmacokinetics. This figure illustrates plasma concentrations following oral administration of a representative NSAID. At any one time, the plasma value reflects the independent contributions of 3 overlapping processes: absorption, distribution, and elimination. NSAIDs generally share similar rates of absorption and distribution but differ in their elimination kinetics.

some sustained-release preparations is to attain steady plasma levels as a result of a constant absorption rate equal to the concurrent rate of elimination. This ideal, 'zero-order kinetics', is probably never attained but may be approached using agents with a long half-life.

Distribution

During the distribution phase of standard plasma pharmacokinetics, the concentration of free drug is greater in plasma than in extravascular interstitial fluid. The resultant concentration gradient drives net diffusion of drug into the surrounding interstitial space. The distribution process is thus one of equilibration of free drug throughout the entire extracellular space (see p.74). Since virtually all NSAIDs bind highly to plasma albumin, the total level of drug (bound plus free) in plasma will exceed that of the normal interstitium at equilibrium because of the corresponding disparity in the concentration of albumin.

Elimination

The final, and most variable, phase of NSAID pharmacokinetics is that of drug metabolism and excretion. For the most part, these agents follow classic first-order kinetics. This means that a constant fraction of available drug is excreted per unit of time (for instance 10%/hour). When the natural log of the drug concentration is plotted against time (as in fig 5.1), drug elimination may be represented by a straight line whose slope (k) is a rate constant. Using the simple formula $t_{1/2} = 0.693/k$, such constants may be converted to a more clinically familiar value: the half-life. Published values for NSAID half-lives vary from the relatively few minutes of aspirin to the days of phenylbutazone.

Several experimental problems should be kept in mind before half-life values are uncritically accepted. When the half-life is short and absorption is prolonged, it may prove difficult to dissociate absorption from elimination. In fact, this may be virtually impossible when the problem is complicated by enterohepatic circulation as it is, for instance, in the case of indomethacin. A further problem ensues from the fact that elimination is rarely so simple as a direct renal excretion of the unchanged parent NSAID. These agents are primarily converted to glucuronides and/or additional metabolites by the liver before they are excreted in the urine. A given half-life value may thus reflect the sum of several different processes and the elimination of more than one product. Different investigators may arrive at quite different values for the half-life of a drug depending on the time period over which they calculate k, the mode of drug administration, the specificity of the method for measuring the parent compound, and the individuals selected for study. For virtually all NSAIDs, pharmacokinetic studies have revealed marked differences between normal subjects in the rates of elimination. Some of this variation results from genetic differences in relevant enzyme systems and from a trend towards impaired elimination in older subjects. For the most part, however, we do not understand the reasons for these critical differences in the rates of drug metabolism and excretion.

Although we now recognize that metabolic variation leads to prominent differences in NSAID concentrations, clinicians are not yet able to recognize and allow for such variations in the management of individual patient problems. Plasma NSAID levels (free and total) can be determined but are generally available only as a tool of selective research studies. Wider access to such methods might well have the same impact on medical care that we have already seen from monitoring of digitalis and phenytoin plasma levels.

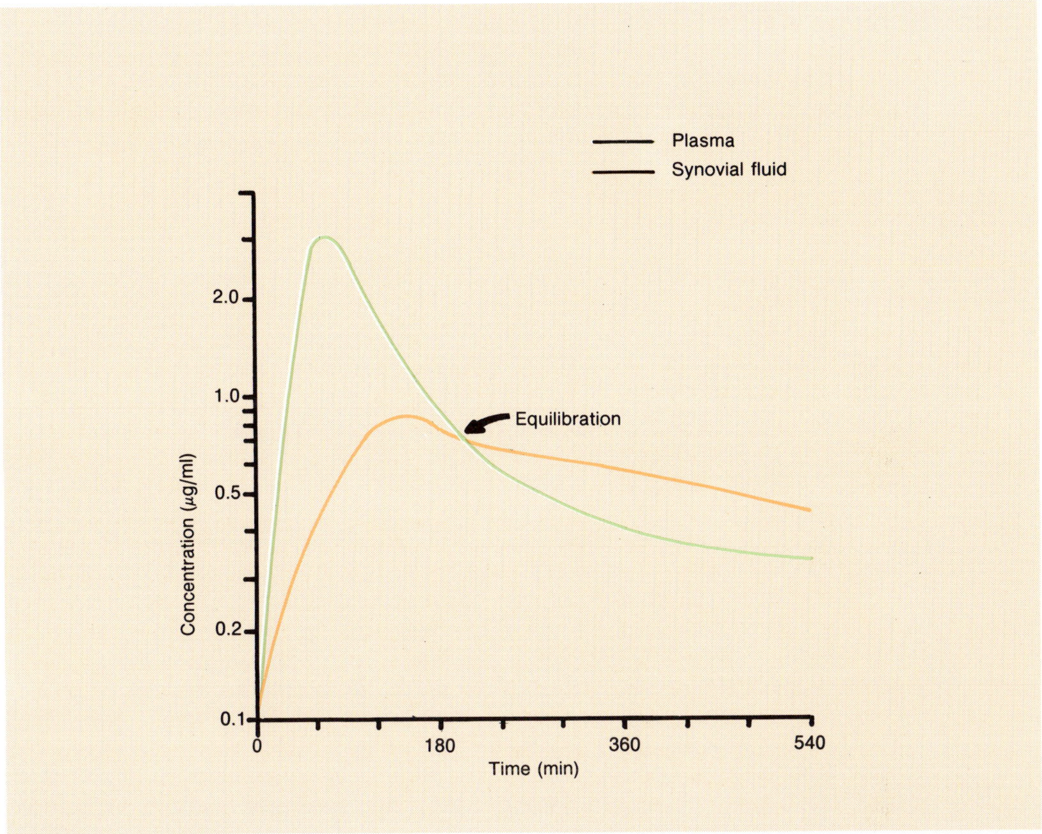

Fig. 5.2. Synovial fluid pharmacokinetics. Synovial fluid concentrations lag behind those in plasma during absorption and distribution. After distribution is complete, however, NSAID levels in synovial fluid (and presumably in other interstitial fluids) exceed those of plasma. Thus, an initial gradient drives net diffusion from blood to tissue. After a specific equilibration time, however, the gradient is reversed and drugs diffuse from the interstitium back into the plasma. (Reproduced with the kind permission of Lea and Febiger).

Practical Application of Half-life Values

Despite the limitations of published half-life determinations, such values have come to play a prominent role in therapeutic decision-making. For the most part, this has been manifested by patient and physician preference for the greater convenience of longer-lived agents. Because of their slow turnover, such drugs need to be taken less often. They are less bother to the patient, whose compliance is therefore likely to be better than with alternative regimens employing frequent doses of short-acting agents.

Stable plasma NSAID levels may not always be necessary. Maintenance of continuous therapy seems most desirable to combat equally continuous levels of inflammatory stimuli. Here, however, we are often handicapped by uncertainty as to the underlying mechanisms of rheumatic diseases. When signs and symptoms occur around the clock, then continuous coverage clearly seems desirable. On the other hand, periodic signs of inflammation related, for instance, to physical activity or to the time of day may be treated most logically with intermittent administration of relatively short-acting agents.

Synovial Fluid Kinetics

Several agents with relatively short half-lives have been promoted on the basis of synovial fluid drug levels higher than those found concurrently in plasma. These experimental findings, however, seem unlikely to reflect any specific therapeutic advantage. As already described, and depicted in figure 5.1, the distribution phase of plasma pharmacokinetics is marked by diffusion gradients from relatively high levels in microvascular plasma to lower concentrations in surrounding interstitial fluid. Pathologic synovial effusions represent a special case which enables sampling of the interstitial fluid in inflamed tissue.

Plotting the intrasynovial drug levels together with concurrent plasma concentrations thus allows direct assessment of the initial gradients favoring drug distribution. Once distribution has been completed, the elimination of drug from plasma creates a reverse gradient driving the free drug back from the interstitium into the perfusing plasma. After each single dose of medication, there is a specific 'equilibration point' which marks the transition between distribution and clearance of that agent (fig 5.2). Ideally, this point should be determined from measurements of free rather than total (free plus protein-bound) drug concentrations. In practice, very few such data are available. This distinction may not be critical, however, in evaluating pathologic effusions of relatively high albumin content.

Clearly, those agents which are cleared rapidly from the plasma would be expected to have early equilibration points leading to their rapid clearance from tissues as well. Conversely, drugs having slower half-lives would be expected to remain longer in tissues as well as in plasma. Just such a relationship was found when equilibration points were estimated, from a number of published studies of synovial fluid NSAID kinetics, and were plotted against plasma half-lives (fig 5.3) [Wallis and Simkin, 1983].

In clinical practice, NSAIDs are rarely given in the single doses used in the studies summarized above. Frequent doses of short-lived drugs may be expected to produce a 'picket fence profile' of rapidly rising and falling drug levels both in plasma and in synovial fluid. Slowly cleared drugs will provide much more gradual fluctuations both in plasma and in tissue levels. Before each dose, the intrasynovial levels of free drug will exceed those of plasma on either program. The less pronounced swings of long half-life drugs will usually mean that the total level of these highly protein-bound agents will remain higher in plasma than in concurrent samples of synovial fluid. There is no clear evidence of more effective suppression of inflammation when fluctuations around the mean drug level are either large or small. Therapeutic choices, therefore, should be based not on synovial fluid levels but on other considerations including cost, convenience and the likelihood of patient compliance.

Short Term or Continuous NSAID Use

Although the preceding discussion reviews a number of aspects of NSAID pharmacokinetics in plasma and in tissues, it does not reveal specific features which would bear on issues of either toxicity or effectiveness. Clearly, one relevant consideration must be the consideration of pharmacokinetics in the selection of agents to treat both chronic and acute inflammatory conditions. The situation is not dissimilar from the use of digitalis in the management of congestive heart failure. Chronic, low-grade symptoms may be man-

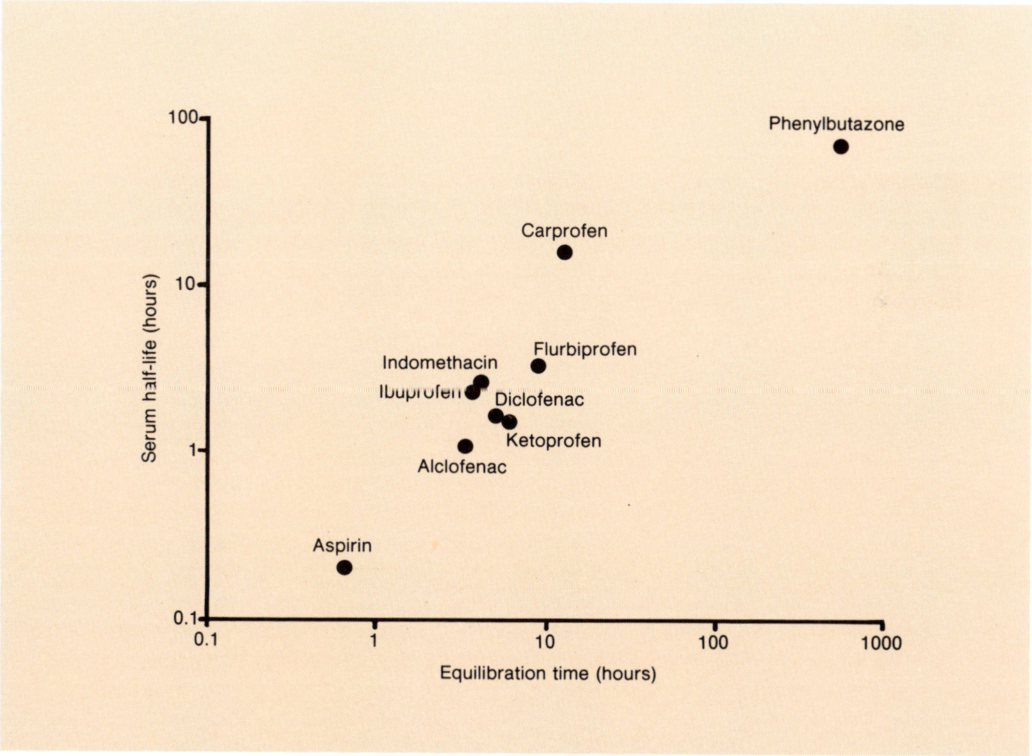

Fig. 5.3. NSAID equilibration time: a function of plasma kinetics. Plasma half-lives are plotted against estimated synovial equilibration times in this figure composed from published data for 9 different NSAIDs (Wallis and Simkin, 1983). Short-lived drugs have only a brief period when the plasma concentration exceeds that of synovial fluid. This property, however, conveys no obvious therapeutic advantage.

aged by starting maintenance therapy and evaluating the response at leisure. Acute pulmonary edema, however, must be recognized as an emergency and managed aggressively. In the same way, acute inflammation deserves an agent and administration regimen which will promptly achieve therapeutic levels in plasma and tissues.

In general, plasma levels of any oral drug will not stabilize until 4 to 5 half-lives of maintenance therapy have gone by. After this point, the plasma concentration will fluctuate around a constant mean value. In treating chronic conditions with long-lived drugs such as piroxicam, the importance of this point lies in ensuring that an adequate trial is given. Uninformed patients may prematurely conclude that the drug is ineffective before baseline plasma levels have been attained. Generally, any slow turnover agent should be tried for at least 2 weeks before one considers alternative measures. Clinical improvement within this period may well progress further during subsequent, sustained therapy. Such a leisurely approach is clearly inappropriate in the management of more emergent inflammatory conditions such as acute gouty arthritis. In such a situation, the physician must choose either high maintenance doses of a short-lived therapeutic agent or loading plus maintenance doses of a long-lived drug.

Pharmacokinetics in Practice

Salicylates as an Example

For the most part, the clearance phase of NSAID pharmacokinetics is reasonably described in terms of straightforward, first-order kinetics. The most striking exception to this rule is the first and, to many, still the foremost class of NSAIDs: the salicylates. These compounds are cleared as 5 different compounds at vastly different kinetic rates. The non-linearity of this aggregate process is demonstrated by one finding that the elimination half-life of low dose salicylate (1.6 mmol) was 2.4h but that of high dose therapy (125 mmol) was 19h (Levy, 1979). This dramatic difference clearly demonstrates a critical role for some process which does not follow first-order kinetics.

The unusual kinetics of salicylate elimination are now known to result from saturation of the system which conjugates salicylate with glycine to form salicyluric acid. Below saturation, the reaction follows typical first-order kinetics. Above that point, however, salicylurate forms at a constant rate regardless of the driving concentration of salicylate ions. Since salicylurate is the predominant excretion product, overall elimination becomes a progressively smaller fraction of the body store as the salicylate level rises. The salicylate half-life, of course, becomes correspondingly longer.

These observations carry critical implications for the therapeutic use of any salicylate preparation. Plasma salicylate levels in the therapeutic range (usually considered to be 20 to 30 mg/dl) are well above the point where salicylurate formation has been saturated. This means that additional dosage increments will lead to a disproportionate rise in salicylate level with a corresponding increase in the risk of toxicity. Thus, for instance, patients who have progressively and uneventfully, escalated their salicylate dosage to 4200 mg/day may experience a marked improvement from a further increase to 4800mg but may suffer severe toxicity at 5400mg. Such a history is not the exception but the rule in using these agents. Fortunately, plasma salicylate levels are widely available to practicing clinicians and such determinations may be valuable both in determining the most appropriate dosage and in ensuring the adequacy of a therapeutic trial. Once the appropriate total dosage has been determined, the prolonged half-life at this level also means that dosage regimens may be selected which best suit the convenience of the patient. In most cases, this means that twice-daily administration is both reasonable and appropriate. No salicylate need be given 4-hourly for the chronic therapy of any rheumatic condition.

Although salicylurate excretion provides the principal path for salicylate clearance, other routes also deserve mention. The simplest and most im-

Table 5.1. Selected pharmacokinetic and chemical properties of commonly used non-steroidal anti-inflammatory drugs

Drug	Usual daily dose (adults) [mg]	Elimination half-life (h)	pKa	Volume of distribution (L/kg)	Plasma protein binding (%)
Salicylates					
Aspirin	3000-6000	0.25	3.5	0.15	> 90
Salicylic acid	3000-6000	2-30	2.95	0.17	80-90
Diflunisal	500-750	5-20	4.0	0.10	> 99
Propionic acid derivatives					
Ibuprofen	1200-2400	2	5.2		99
Naproxen	500-1000	12-15	4.2	0.10	< 99
Fenoprofen	1200-2400	2-3	4.5	0.10	< 99
Indole derivatives					
Indomethacin	75-150	5-10	5.3	0.15-0.20	> 90
Sulindac	300-400	7-16	4.7		93
Tolmetin	800-1200	1-1.5	3.5	0.10-0.14	> 99
Pyrazoles					
Phenylbutazone[a]	300-400	50-100	4.5	0.17	98-99
Oxyphenbutazone[b]	300-400	27-64			98-99
Fenamates					
Mefenamic acid	1500	3-4	4.33		High
Meclofenamate	200-400	3	2.30		> 99
Oxicams					
Piroxicam	20	31-57	6.3	0.12-0.14	> 99

a Phenylbutazone is no longer available in the UK except for treating ankylosing spondylitis in hospitalized patients.
b Recently withdrawn in the UK.

portant of these is direct clearance of the unchanged salicylate ion. Although this is a first-order process, its rate varies markedly as a function of urinary pH.

Non-polar, unionized salicylate diffuses out of renal tubules when the urine is acidic and salicylate clearance is correspondingly low. On urinary alkalinization however, the salicylate remains both ionized and intratubular. Clearance may be increased 20-fold by raising the pH from 5.0 to 8.0. At this point, salicylate ion excretion becomes an important clearance mechanism thus earning the time-honored place for alkalinization in the therapy of salicylate intoxication.

The other excretion forms of salicylate are 2 glucuronides (salicyl- and salicyl phenolic-) and the oxidation product: gentisic acid. Of these metabolites, salicyl phenolic glucuronide also has a saturable formation system analogous to that of salicylurate. Knowledge of these products has greatly helped to complete the story of salicylate metabolism. The clinician reader, however, need consider these minor products no further.

Other Drugs

Further exceptions to the rule of simple kinetics for NSAIDs are found in sulindac and in fenbufen. Both of these agents are prodrugs which do not become active until they are metabolized to their active products. In both cases, however, these active products may then be reasonably characterized in terms of first-order kinetics.

The principal pharmacokinetic properties of some of the more common NSAIDs are listed in table 5.1 together with the chemical properties to be discussed below. Details of structure and classification have not been repeated since these points are discussed by Dr Klinenberg in chapter 1. The present list is not inclusive but has been selected to illustrate the range of properties among NSAIDs now in common use.

Chemical Properties

Organic Acidity

The consistent carboxylic acid moiety of NSAIDs bears no specific relationship to the beneficial activity of these agents but may be critical to their most important form of toxicity: the significant risk of gastritis and ulcer. From mild dyspepsia to catastrophic hemorrhage, the range of gastric side effects (see chapter 4, p.60) provides the principal limiting factor in the administration of aspirin and of essentially every other available NSAID. It is important to note that these risks are predominantly gastric. There is much less evidence of significant toxicity to the duodenum or to subsequent portions of the small or large intestine. Both anecdotal and systematic observations suggest that large particle size and relative insolubility of tablets both contribute to the likelihood of NSAID-induced gastric lesions. Conversely, endoscopic studies indicate that gastric risk is greatly diminished or eliminated when comparable

NSAID dosage is administered intravenously or by rectal suppository. Such findings suggest that local gastric toxicity provides the greatest contribution to the gastrointestinal complications of NSAID therapy. It is this local gastric toxicity which appears to be related to the fact that NSAIDs are weak organic acids.

Local Gastric Toxicity

The best evidence of local gastric toxicity comes from Davenport's classical studies of aspirin in the canine stomach (Davenport, 1967). This work demonstrated several critical findings:

1) Intragastric aspirin causes cytotoxic changes in mucosal cells, interruption of the mucosal barrier, and induction of erosive lesions in the submucosa.

2) These changes can be prevented by introducing the same amount of aspirin in a neutral buffer.

3) Distension of the stomach significantly increases the risk of submucosal lesions.

These observations are best interpreted within the context of a hypothesis beginning with the fact that aspirin is a weak organic acid having a pKa of 2.95 (Martin, 1963). At pH levels above this point the acid dissociates and exists as highly polar aspirin ions. Below a pH of 2.3, on the other hand, aspirin exists predominantly as the undissociated acid. In this form, aspirin can diffuse across the bilayer lipid membrane of gastric lining cells just as it does within the renal tubule. Within the cell, aspirin again dissociates at the relatively high pH of normal cytoplasm and the agent may thus be trapped within the mucosal cell. Because of the presence of ingested aspirin immediately adjacent to the mucosal lining, it seems reasonable to presume that gastric cellular concentrations of aspirin reach levels far greater than those found in any other cell. This discretely localized salicylism would be toxic to the cells involved with resultant deformation and disruption of the mucosal barrier. This disruption, in turn, would permit access of gastric acid and enzymes to submucosal tissue where secondary erosive changes would ensue. Distension of the stomach might enhance the transport of gastric juice across the damaged mucosal barrier thereby promoting submucosal injury (fig. 5.4).

The most critical finding supporting this extended hypothesis is the fact that the lesions may be prevented by maintaining a gastric pH at a level higher than the pKa of the offending organic acid. Since the other members of the NSAID group share the property of being weak organic acids and the propensity for gastric injury, it seems reasonable to suggest that they also share a mechanism similar to the gastric cellular salicylism which Martin has suggested for aspirin (Martin, 1963).

Once within the cell, salicylate and other NSAIDs might impair gastric mucosal defenses by one or more of several possible mechanisms. Direct cellular cytotoxicity, as originally postulated by Martin, remains a very real possibility through interference with protein synthesis, uncoupling of oxidative phosphorylation, impaired cyclic AMP metabolism, or similar metabolic interference. More appealing, however, is the concept that gastric toxicity is me-

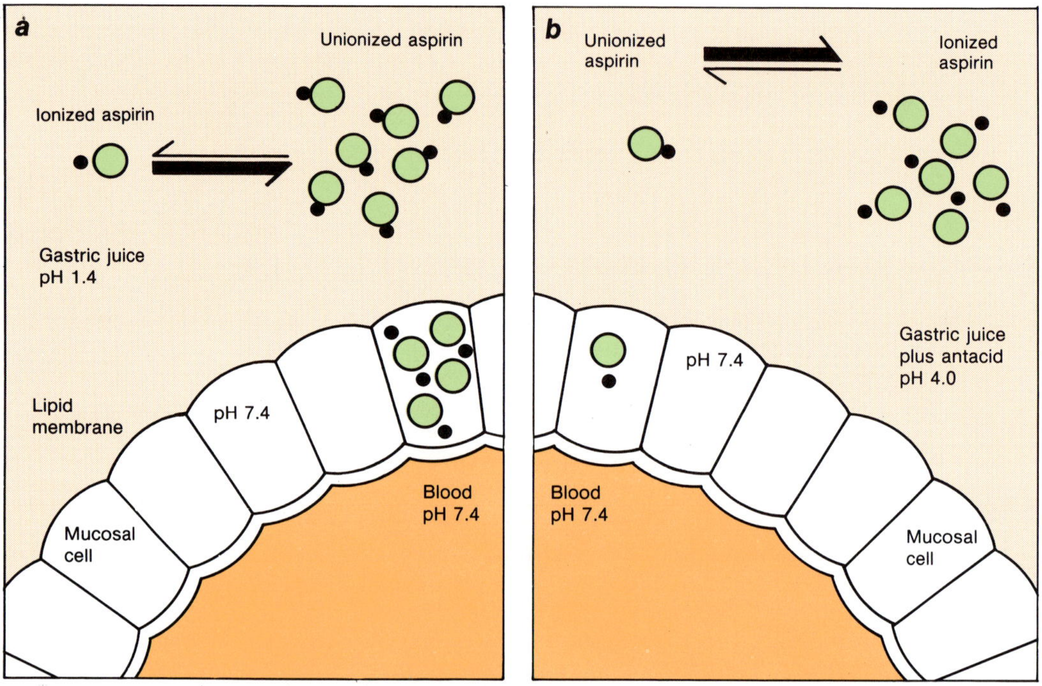

Fig. 5.4. Diagrammatic representation of the Martin hypothesis. **a)** In gastric juice at pH 1.4 aspirin is present largely in unionized form which readily diffuses across the lipid membrane. Once inside the mucosal cell at pH 7.4 it ionizes and can then leave the cell only as it again becomes unionized. **b)** Raising the pH above the pKa leaves the aspirin largely ionized and thus unable to enter the mucosal cell.

diated locally by the best known property of these agents: inhibition of prostaglandin synthesis. Substantial evidence now indicates that exogenous as well as endogenous prostaglandins possess significant 'cytoprotective properties which serve to defend the gastric mucosa against the ever-present hazard of autodigestion. Inhibition of such defenses would obviously expose the stomach to increased risks of gastritis and erosion. Regardless of the mechanism of NSAID toxicity, however, long-standing evidence suggests that the stomach will be protected if the ingested drugs do not diffuse into mucosal cells.

Practical Application

The greatest virtue of the Martin hypothesis is that it defines a critical pathologic process and at the same time suggests a simple and logical prophylactic plan. The way to avoid mucosal injury from aspirin would seem to be to ensure that the drug is never present in an acidic stomach. The easiest, and least expensive way to achieve this goal is to administer the agent with antacid approximately half an hour or more *before* meals. At this time, the stomach has not been stimulated to produce gastric acid and enzymes, gastric emptying has not been delayed by ingestion of proteins and fat, and the stomach has not been distended by a meal. It is at this time that a modest dose of oral antacid is most likely to achieve its goal of gastric neutralization and that the offending drug can be moved on into the small intestine without the special risk to mucosal cells caused by unionized, non-polar aspirin within the gastric lumen.

Alternative approaches, including effective enteric coating, less soluble forms of salicylate, and (to a degree) admixture of buffering agents, have already served to reduce the gastric risk of long term therapy with aspirin and other salicylates.

A number of important lessons remain, however, which may pertain not only to salicylate but to the other weak organic acids among the NSAID family. Foremost among these is the concept that such agents should not be taken after meals when the stomach is distended, gastric emptying is delayed, and the rate of mucosal acid production is at its highest point. Sadly, it is at just this time that many dyspeptic patients are advised to ingest these potentially toxic compounds. In the author's experience, most patients can comfortably ingest virtually any NSAID before meals with a modest dose of antacid.

Physicians contemplating such a program should be aware that antacid intake sufficient to neutralize or alkalinize the urine will increase the renal clearance of salicylate and might do so as well for other weak organic acids (see also chapter 4, p.66). In addition, this administration scheme will in no way ameliorate the potential enteric risk of diminished systemic prostaglandin synthesis. Nonetheless, the great majority of dyspeptic NSAID users may show a substantial net benefit from this mode of administration.

Protein Binding – Its Clinical Implications

A second, shared 'chemical' property of available NSAIDs is a high degree of reversible binding to plasma proteins (table 5.1). More specifically, these agents bind to albumin. We have already seen that this property leads to a higher NSAID concentration in microvascular plasma than in the surrounding interstitial fluid (p.75). The low apparent distribution volume of these drugs (table 5.1) reflects both this high degree of intravascular binding to plasma proteins and the absence of significant extravascular binding in peripheral tissues.

The clinical consequences of protein binding appear to be of rather limited significance (McElnay and D'Arcy, 1983). Hypoalbuminemia, an occasional finding in rheumatoid disease, may result in somewhat lower total concentrations but would not be expected to alter availability of the free drug. Were NSAIDs all to bind to the same site on plasma albumin, the finding would carry the intriguing implication of a shared molecular configuration which might underly some of the therapeutic benefits and toxic risks which these agents have in common. In fact, however, a number of different binding sites appear to be involved and salicylate ions, for instance, can bind to more than one site per albumin molecule.

Competition does occur between NSAIDs for the same apparent binding site but on the whole such interaction is as impressive for its absence as for its presence. Certainly there are no convincing grounds to believe that competitive displacement of one NSAID by another is likely to increase the toxic risk (or diminish the therapeutic benefit) of concurrently administered agents above that of either drug given alone (at correspondingly increased dosage).

There is reason for concern, however, over the possibility that other therapeutic agents may be potentiated by abrupt displacement from binding sites on serum albumin. So far, the most convincing examples of such interactions involve the effects of oxyphenbutazone and phenylbutazone on plasma levels of oral anticoagulants (see chapter 4, table 4.1). Patients taking warfarin or related agents should be monitored closely if it becomes necessary or desirable to institute therapy with NSAIDs. Conversely, however, naproxen, mefenamic acid, ketoprofen, and ibuprofen do not appear to potentiate the effects of oral anticoagulant therapy (McElnay and D'Arcy, 1983). Physicians prescribing such agents must still be aware, however, of the platelet inhibition common to all of these drugs (see also chapter 4, p.64).

In considering the protein binding properties of NSAIDs, it has generally been assumed that only the free drug is pharmacologically active. This assumption need not be true. Another highly bound weak organic acid, para-amino hippurate, is carried in such a manner that essentially all of this agent is recognized and excreted during each passage of plasma past proximal renal tubules of normal persons. In this case, protein binding may 'present' this agent to relatively specific cellular receptors. Were such a mechanism to be operative for NSAIDs, the exposed rather than the bound portion of each molecule might carry the structural characteristics critical for pharmacologic and possibly for toxic effects. There is little direct support for this hypothesis. It remains important, however, to consider all such possibilities carefully until the molecular mechanisms of NSAID actions have been established.

Inhibition of Prostaglandin Synthesis – Its Consequences, Good and Bad

Among the properties shared by NSAIDs, none is better known than the ability to inhibit the production of prostaglandins by cyclo-oxygenase enzymes (see chapter 2, p.15). Largely through the widely recognized and nobly nobly rewarded studies of Vane this action has been accepted as the principal mechanism by which these agents inhibit inflammation (Vane, 1971). The broad spectrum of clinical and experimental conditions which respond to NSAIDs has played a major role in establishing the pre-eminent position of prostaglandins among the myriad of mediators known today. Conversely, the apparent importance of prostaglandin inhibition has clearly contributed to the emergence and growth of the NSAID industry.

Does it Correlate with Therapeutic Effectiveness?

Not surprisingly, considerable effort has been devoted to correlations between objective measurements of prostaglandin inhibition and clinical indices of NSAID effectiveness. For the most part, these efforts have been disappointing. The principal problem appears to lie in the substantial differences between species and between tissues in the same species (Metz, 1981). Comparable concentrations of selected NSAIDs may cause quite different responses in seemingly similar models of inflammation. These distinctions should make sense when we have a better understanding of the roles of specific prostaglandins in different forms of clinical and experimental inflammation. Until then, there can be no 'gold standard' of prostaglandin inhibition to be used in ranking the therapeutic effectiveness of available NSAIDs.

Influence on Gastric Toxicity

The record is somewhat better when local NSAID toxicity is correlated with prostaglandin levels in the affected tissues. Perhaps the best example of such work is that of Rainsford with gastric ulcer models both in the pig and in the rat (Rainsford, 1982). These studies appear to demonstrate that the agents and doses most likely to induce gastric ulceration are also those most likely to reduce mucosal levels of prostaglandins. Unfortunately, such a correlation does not establish cause and effect. Gastric lesions and prostaglandin depletion could both result from other cytotoxic NSAID properties.

Other Effects

There is little reason to doubt that inhibition of prostaglandin synthesis is and will remain the most important therapeutic property of the NSAID class. The very multitude of such drugs, however, has now begun to focus attention not on this dominant property, which NSAIDs share, but on the other effects which may serve to distinguish them.

Before the discovery of prostaglandins, textbooks of pharmacology included lengthy lists of the properties of aspirin. Many of these disparate effects now seem attributable to the multiple physiologic roles of prostaglandins, but others remain as specific properties of aspirin or as broader characteristics of the salicylate class. It is presumably from among such secondary characteristics that the subtle distinctions emerge which lead specific NSAIDs to differ in their effectiveness against different rheumatic diseases or among individual patients with the same condition. The next frontier of NSAID development clearly seems directed toward control not only of prostaglandins but also of the lipoxygenase pathway, of free radicals, of the various cytokines, of immunologic processes and doubtless of other mechanisms yet to be established.

Just as secondary properties seem likely to distinguish between the therapeutic benefits of NSAIDs, so also do they appear most responsible for the more selective toxic effects. Headaches, tinnitus, diarrhea, photosensitivity, and other less common reactions occur predominantly among patients taking specific agents (see chapter 4). In such cases, it may be most difficult to define a molecular mechanism of toxicity.

Renal Compromise

Among the toxic reactions suffered by NSAID users, perhaps the most dangerous is that of abrupt renal compromise on institution of therapy. This problem has been studied extensively and now seems to be clearly secondary to NSAID inhibition of prostaglandin synthesis. When renal function has been impaired by any of a number of chronic conditions, the kidney appears to respond with the synthesis and release of prostaglandins to maintain a functional renal blood flow. Disruption of this sustaining system occasionally leads to acute renal failure in patients who previously had enjoyed a stable and satisfactory level of renal function. This catastrophic complication is perhaps the best example in which the intended result (inhibition of prostaglandin synthesis) turns out to worsen rather than to alleviate the patient's overall condition.

Encouraging evidence suggests that such untoward renal effects may be partially bypassed by employing the prodrug: sulindac. The agent with the NSAID activity is not sulindac itself but its sulfide metabolite. Any tissue lacking the appropriate enzymes to cleave this drug might thus be expected to be free of either its beneficial or its toxic properties. The impaired kidney may be such a deficient tissue. The stomach, however, is not and this prodrug does not appear to have less gastric toxicity than do many other available NSAIDs (Rainsford, 1982). For the most part, it seems unreasonable to expect that effective prodrugs will be found which are enzymatically activated only at sites of inflammation and not in normal tissues.

Salicylate Hypersensitivity

An interesting reaction occurring among some but not all non-steroidal agents is the classic asthmatic episode of salicylate hypersensitivity. The allergic nature of these episodes suggest an antigen shared by these drugs alone or as haptens on carrier proteins. If the immunologic recognition were of the active site of the drug, this unfortunate reaction could provide a most useful tool for the molecular definition of important NSAID members. Such speculation, of course, would require extensive investigative work before its possible value could be fairly evaluated.

Structure-Activity Relationships

Non-steroidal anti-inflammatory drugs are all the same but are somehow different. Which one is best and how can it be made better? These questions at present consume much of the time and effort of the best pharmaceutical chemists in the world (Shen, 1981). Their attempts to decipher the structure-activity relationships of NSAIDs have led to more and more molecular modifications many of which have found a role in therapy and thus in the pharmaceutical marketplace. Unfortunately, none of the new drugs is so superior that it has rendered older agents obsolete. There clearly is reason to hope, however, that continued evolution will give us not just more and different agents but also clearly superior agents.

The starting point, at present, is the structure of those available agents which have been found to inhibit prostaglandin synthesis. Unfortunately, drug molecules are not laid out like this page, in two dimensions as shown in figure 1.4, but are complex three-dimensional structures. Published diagrams of molecular configurations thus do little justice to the similarities and differences in the design of useful NSAIDs. The more appropriate three-dimensional models may be viewed as a series of imperfect keys from which the medicinal chemist attempts to design a better key but only to open a lock whose inner workings remain unseen. As yet, we have little knowledge of the biological sites where drug molecules act. Such information is crucial to the molecular understanding not only of structure-function relationships in effective therapy but also of structure-dysfunction interactions underlying drug toxicity.

References

Davenport, H.W.: Salicylate damage to the gastric mucosal barrier. New England Journal of Medicine 276: 1307-1312 (1967).

Levy, G.: Pharmacokinetics of salicylate in man. Drug Metabolism Reviews 9: 3-19 (1979).

Martin, B.K.: Accumulation of drug anions in gastric mucosal cells. Nature 198: 896-897 (1963).

McElnay, J.C. and D'Arcy, P.F.: Protein binding displacement interactions and their clinical importance. Drugs 25: 495-513 (1983).

Metz, S.A.: Anti-inflammatory agents as inhibitors of prostaglandin synthesis in man. Medical Clinics of North America 65: 713-757 (1981).

Rainsford, K.D.: An analysis of the gastro-intestinal side effects of non-steroidal anti-inflammatory drugs, with particular reference to comparative studies in man and laboratory species. Rheumatology International 2: 1-10 (1982).

Shen, T.Y.: Toward more selective antiarthritic therapy. Journal of Medicinal Chemistry 24: 1-5 (1981).

Vane, J.R.: Inhibition of prostaglandin synthesis as a mechanism of action for aspirin-like drugs. Nature (New Biology) 231: 232-235 (1971).

Verbeeck, R.K.; Blackburn, J.L. and Loewen, G.R.: Clinical pharmacokinetics of non-steroidal anti-inflammatory drugs. Clinical Pharmacokinetics 8: 297-331 (1983).

Wallis, W.J. and Simkin, P.A.: Antirheumatic drug concentrations in human synovial fluid and synovial tissue observations on extravascular pharmacokinetics. Clinical Pharmacokinetics 8: 496-522 (1983).

6. Dosage Regimens and Dose Form Modification

J.M.H. Moll

Sheffield Centre for Rheumatic Diseases, Nether Edge Hospital, Sheffield, England

This chapter is largely intended to examine aspects of handling NSAIDs in clinical practice, and in particular will include comments on dosage regimens from the point of view of amount, frequency and timing of doses. Additional comments have been included on related areas – reformulations, compliance, the use of NSAIDs as analgesics, and NSAIDs in relation to future needs.

The comments are largely based on United Kingdom experience and the drug listings are entirely based on those used in the United Kingdom (see chapter 1, table 1.1).

Intrinsic Activity

Is There a Justification for 'Minor' and 'Major' NSAIDs?

Most NSAIDs have been shown to be effective anti-inflammatory drugs in rheumatoid arthritis. The usual comparisons have been to test new NSAIDs against either placebo or aspirin (see chapter 2, p.28). However, relatively few studies have compared the newer agents with each other. In the context of regular arguments concerning whether or not it is justifiable to classify NSAIDs into those with 'minor' and 'major' effects, any studies in this area are of interest.

Huskisson et al. (1976) and Reynolds and Whorwell (1974) found that naproxen was the most effective of the several NSAIDs they tested. In another comparative study involving propionic acid derivatives, Gall et al. (1982) found that naproxen, fenoprofen, ibuprofen and tolmetin were better tolerated than aspirin, but of similar anti-inflammatory efficacy. However, in terms of the ranking of patients' and physicians' preferences (as opposed to evaluation in terms of statistical significances), the order of preference was the same as in previous studies: naproxen, ibuprofen, fenoprofen, tolmetin, aspirin. In a further study of rheumatoid patients – an Australasian 10-centre group study (Australasian Multicentre Trial Group, 1980) of 400 subjects – naproxen, ibuprofen, sulindac, salicylates and placebo were compared. All active agents were found to be more effective than placebo, but not significantly different from one another.

Wasner et al. (1981) conducted a trial in 33 patients with rheumatoid arthritis and 32 with ankylosing spondylitis. Six NSAIDs were tested in a double-blind randomized crossover study with 6 weeks on each drug. Naproxen, indomethacin and fenoprofen proved to be the most effective drugs in ankylosing spondylitis, whilst in rheumatoid arthritis there was little difference in effect between the drugs.

From present evidence, limited though it is, there would appear to be little justification in dividing NSAIDs into minor and major drugs. However, it is generally believed that there are small differences in anti-inflammatory activity between the drugs, with aspirin, indomethacin and phenylbutazone representing the most potent NSAIDs and the rest, notably propionic acid preparations such as naproxen, falling only a little behind (if at all) in terms of efficacy. Nevertheless, the fact that many of these newer agents will control acute gout testifies to their significant anti-inflammatory effect.

Dosage According to Predominant Symptoms

NSAIDs possess both analgesic and anti-inflammatory properties. In disorders in which the inflammatory component is relatively mild, such as in osteoarthritis, smaller dosages of NSAIDs are usually sufficient to control pain, stiffness and swelling; and when pain alone is the problem, a plain analgesic without anti-inflammatory effects is effective in controlling symptoms. When the inflammatory changes are more prominent, as in rheumatoid arthritis or the disorders of the spondarthritis group, maximal maintenance dosages may be needed. Within these disorders, however, there is a wide range of symptomatic severity, and the aim should always be to use the *smallest dosage* necessary to control symptoms. In individual patients, the level of dosage may have to be varied according to the level of inflammatory activity at any one time. Therefore, within an acceptable range of dosage, the approach is one of 'titrating' the daily amount of drug given to the needs of the patient, rather than prescribing a 'fixed dosage'. In conditions in which the inflammatory component is intense, as in acute gout, the highest acceptable dose will have to be given for a few days to control acute symptoms until the dose can be dropped to a maintenance level.

Supplementary Analgesics

In patients with rheumatoid arthritis and other chronic inflammatory arthritides, NSAIDs may not in themselves provide sufficient analgesic effect, despite their efficacy in suppressing the inflammatory manifestations of the disease. In patients with long-standing disease, secondary degenerative changes may supervene, and these may compound the painful effect of the primary disease. The addition of a plain analgesic [such as acetaminophen (paracetamol)] to NSAID therapy may be useful in these patients to provide additional pain relief. The prescribing of analgesics and NSAIDs as separate drugs is preferable to giving compound analgesic-NSAID preparations, since individual adjustments of either drug can be made if necessary. However, this is only a general rule, and it may be found that the symptomatic relief gained from a compound preparation (e.g. 'Safapryn' = acetaminophen + aspirin; 'Veganin' = acetaminophen + codeine phosphate + aspirin) may, inexplicably, be more effective than the same drugs prescribed individually. Whether this is a 'real' benefit or one based on 'placebo factors', the patient need not be denied a preferred drug given as a compound, as long as the basis for prescribing it is sound.

Amount of Dosing

Patterns of Introducing NSAIDs – Increasing or Decreasing to Maintenance Dosage

The pattern of introducing NSAID therapy may vary according to the condition treated and/or the drug used.

In general, in patients with inflammatory arthritis, and especially when the inflammation is marked, a loading dose is given, after which the dosage is reduced to a maintenance level. This pattern of administration is particularly important in controlling acute gout, and these patients seem to tolerate even 'supramaximal' dosages without side effects – perhaps because the extent of the inflammation 'soaks up' the drug more than when inflammation is of a more subacute type. In osteoarthrosis, however, the importance of achieving maximal blood levels rapidly is not so pressing, and in these patients the starting dose with most NSAIDs can be the maintenance dose. In the treatment of rheumatoid arthritis, the need to prescribe a loading dose will depend on the acuteness of the problem.

Some drugs are best given in a small dosage to start with, in order to reduce the risk of intolerance/rejection. A particular example is indomethacin, which is usually better tolerated if gradually introduced.

Indications for Maximal Dosage

Some aspects of this have already been mentioned. However, the subject merits discussion in further detail.

The term 'maximal dosage' should be interpreted flexibly, within sensible constraints imposed by the manufacturers' recommendations, and there should be an appreciation of the meaning of maximal dosage for short periods (a few days) and for maintenance. The maximal dosage for a frail, elderly woman will doubtless not be the maximal dose for a hefty young man, although the 'maximum' recorded in standard reference works will usually be expressed as a single value. Indeed, there may be a considerable difference in response to a particular drug between two individuals of similar build. Laurence (1973) has stressed that when a patient is given a drug the response is the resultant of several factors in addition to the pharmacodynamic effect of the drug, and that these factors may lead to the modification of

Table 6.1. Factors that may affect the response of patients to a given dosage of an NSAID and which may necessitate individual dosage adjustment

Interactions with any other drug the patient may be taking
The physiological state of the end-organ – whether, for example, it is over- or underactive
The act of medication, including the route of administration, and the presence or absence of the doctor
The doctor's mood, personality, attitudes and beliefs
What the doctor has told the patient
The patient's past experience of doctors
The patient's estimate of treatment received and what ought to be the outcome
The social environment, e.g. whether the patient is alone or in company

what should be regarded as the maximum dose. Some of these factors are outlined in table 6.1.

Varying Dosage within Maintenance Range

Chronic inflammatory arthritides whether of rheumatoid, spondarthritic or other 'idiopathic' types, are characterized by unpredictable fluctuations in inflammatory activity. The dosage of NSAID will therefore need to be varied according to these clinical changes. This can be done by the family practitioner or by the rheumatologist at review. However, this arrangement may deny the patient a few days or weeks of benefit from a higher dose (in the case of arthritis in relapse) or cause the needless ingestion of maximal doses (when the arthritis enters a phase of remission). Adequate communication with the patient should enable many to adjust their own dosages according to how they feel. This, of course, may not be feasible in patients who have difficulty in understanding, seeing or hearing. However, in most instances careful verbal explanation supplemented by a written/drawn memorandum should ensure that patients can control their own dosage planning, with supervision from the clinician at suitable intervals.

As mentioned above, the aim should always be to give the smallest possible dose to control the arthritis adequately. In some patients, notably those with ankylosing spondylitis, reasonable control of disease in remission may be achieved by a single tablet daily, or even one tablet on alternate days.

The author advises selected patients who appear to be experiencing significant periods of remission to try discontinuing their tablets for short periods. In doing this it is important to stress the advisability of gradual weaning, rather than suddenly stopping NSAIDs. However, with NSAIDs this principle is not so important as in patients on corticosteroids.

Continuous Versus Interrupted Dosage

In general, patients with rheumatoid arthritis and other 'low-grade' but inexorable chronic arthritides, such as ankylosing spondylitis, will need NSAID medication continuously, albeit as stated above, there may be phases of remission during which the patient can do without treatment.

In some chronic arthropathies the expression of the joint disease is very mild, and continuing dosage is not justified. A good example is psoriatic arthritis in which often only a few joints are involved, often not weight-bearing ones. These patients may be able to manage for months (sometimes years) without medication. However, they will learn to recognize when their disease is entering a phase of relapse, and will then need to restart NSAIDs for a period.

Another example in which interrupted NSAID administration is useful is in patients with only occasional attacks of gout in which the prodromal features are recognizable. These patients, experiencing attacks spaced by one or even several years, can simply dose themselves at the first sign of an impending attack, and discontinue medication after it has settled. Clearly, should episodes become more frequent, regular NSAID treatment or even a long term hypouricemic drug may be necessary.

Interrupted dosage is usually more appropriate than continued medication in patients with recurrent soft tissue lesions. The patients with repeated episodes of tennis elbow, rotator-cuff pain or other short-lived syndromes in the domain of 'medical orthopedics' should not need long term NSAID therapy. These acute episodes usually respond to a short course of NSAID for 2 or 3 weeks, preferably in maximal dosage if this can be tolerated.

Caution in Special Circumstances – Children, the Elderly, the Sick, and the Frail

Under certain circumstances particular care should be taken to ensure that drug dosage is modified to cater for altered physiologic/metabolic requirements. In juveniles, the elderly (see also chapter 3, table 3.1), and those with concomitant illness, or those who are frail and underweight, special caution is necessary.

Children

Baum (1982) has enumerated the following general facts, general rules and ethical principles concerning the use of drugs in children, and one can do no better than to summarize those relevant to NSAID therapy:

1) It is prudent to remember that children are not simply small adults. *Proper dosage levels and side effects cannot be deduced from data obtained from adult studies.*

2) In general, side effects from NSAIDs seem to be fewer in children.

3) A general rule should be that no drug is used in a child until it has been tested and used in adults. Moreover, the medication trials in adults

should preferably last for at least a year to provide adequate opportunity to examine long term as well as short term side effects.

4) Drugs given less often can be a distinct advantage in treating children. Drugs with longer half-lives may therefore be useful for children, as well as for adults.

5) Regarding drug trials in children, the question of age of consent might arise. In Baum's view the parent or guardian should be responsible for providing consent for children below the age of 12. After the age of 12, informed consent should be from the children themselves, as well as from the legal guardians. This approach is supported by the study of Bibace and Walsh (1980) who found that children in the United States have an early realization and understanding of disease in terms of disordered physiology by the age of 11. Below this age, concepts of disease are essentially 'non-physiologic'.

The Elderly

Studies in geriatric patients with arthritis have shown that the elderly are more likely to suffer side effects from drugs than are younger patients. The NSAIDs are no exception to this rule. When prescribing a drug that is largely eliminated via the kidney, the dosage of certain NSAIDs may have to be reduced as renal function is usually reduced in old people (see chapter 3, table 3.1). Special caution will be needed in prescribing for osteoarthritic patients, as they tend to be elderly. Moreover, clinical trials of new NSAIDs should always include elderly patients, as assumptions based on safety in younger people could be dangerous if applied too generally.

Other therapeutic considerations in the elderly concern physical rather than physiologic/metabolic matters. Old people may find difficulty in reading instructions, opening containers, swallowing pills or inserting suppositories; they may also have difficulties in getting prescriptions repeated because of transport or communication problems.

Patients with Concomitant Diseases

Particular attention should be directed to the presence of concomitant illness when prescribing NSAIDs. Some examples are as follows:

1) Prescribe indomethacin with caution in patients with CNS disturbances (e.g. epilepsy, Parkinsonism, psychiatric illness).

2) Prescribe salicylates with caution in patients with allergic diseases (e.g. asthma, angioneurotic edema).

3) Avoid phenylbutazone and related drugs in patients with cardiovascular disease (fluid retention).

4) Avoid mefenamic acid in patients with inflammatory bowel disease.

5) Avoid all NSAIDs when active peptic ulceration is present, and prescribe them with caution in those with a history of such disease.

6) Certain NSAIDs potentiate the effect of hypoglycemics and oral anticoagulants (see chapter 4, p.64). Special care is therefore needed to monitor the effect of any interaction between these drugs by regular blood glucose and prothrombin estimations.

In addition to the above examples involving specific drugs or groups of drugs, patients with malabsorption and/or liver disease may require some modifications of dosage; in malabsorption, the dose may have to be increased, and in liver disease a reduction may be needed (see chapter 3, p.46 and table 3.1).

The Frail

In patients who are considerably below 'ideal' weight, NSAIDs should be prescribed in reduced dosage. Some manufacturers provide special guidance on this (e.g. flufenamic acid should not exceed 10 mg/kg daily in patients less than 45kg).

Frequency of Dosing

Clinical Significance of Dose Frequency

The clinical significance of the daily spacing of drug-taking in rheumatology is based on the inherent diurnal pattern of symptoms in individual rheumatoses. The aim is to ensure that maximal blood levels are achieved when symptoms are at their worst.

Three main patterns are seen:

1) The pattern of low-grade chronic inflammatory arthritis of which rheumatoid arthritis is the most common example. These patients characteristically feel worst first thing in the morning, and pain and stiffness on waking may cause difficulties in getting out of bed, bathing and grooming. During the morning they become more mobile. The duration of the morning stiffness is taken as a reasonable index of the level of inflammatory activity (see chapter 2, p.24).

Patients with ankylosing spondylitis display a similar pattern with marked joint stiffness on waking. These patients may also experience spinal pain during the night, forcing them to get up and walk about. Spondylitic patients, unlike patients with disc disease, are happier when they are up and about and active.

2) The unpredictable spikes of inflammatory activity of gout contrast with the more stable pattern of the arthritides discussed above. In these patients the bad days of the acute episode are usually spaced by weeks, months or years of pain-free existence, unless chronic gouty arthritis has supervened.

3) Degenerative arthritis has another pattern of symptoms. In these disorders immobility stiffness ('gelling') is the over-riding feature, in addition to a deep-seated chronic background pain. These patients are more comfortable when using their joints. In patients with osteoarthritis of the knees, prolonged periods of sitting, such as a bus ride or waiting in the surgery, can cause great discomfort when standing and walking are resumed.

In order to allow for these various patterns of arthritic expression, NSAIDs should be prescribed so that adequate analgesic/anti-inflammatory cover is given at an appropriate time. As will be seen in the next section, there is a wealth of choice of drugs for this purpose - a choice enabled largely by the different half-lives of these products.

Drugs with Different Frequencies of Administration

NSAIDs can be classified according to whether they need to be administered 1, 2, 3 or 4 or more times daily (table 6.2).

In patients in whom symptoms are prominent during the night and on waking, a larger dose can be given on retiring to relieve this. For example, if the NSAID is of the thrice-daily type the dosage pattern in such patients might be Xmg am; Xmg midday; X × 2mg pm (e.g. indomethacin 50mg/50mg/100mg).

This approach should not be too strict, and should be tailored to the needs of individual patients. For example, some patients with inflammatory joint disease actually feel *worse* towards the end of the day and better in the morning.

In general, patients seem to prefer drugs that need only once- or twice-daily administration, and this preference could lead to improved compliance. However, this needs to be further verified in a controlled way.

It appears to the author that there is at least one merit in taking tablets at closer intervals. This concerns the reinforcement of a regular habit ('imprinting') developed while taking drugs several times a day. On this basis, therefore, one could argue that, thus 'programmed', the patient has less chance of forgetting his or her medication.

Nevertheless, the practical value of once-daily administration has been well proven in the field of the contraceptive pill, and one factor may be that if motivation is sufficient, forgetfulness diminishes. However, if the one and only single daily dose is forgotten the loss is obviously greater than if only one of three or four daily doses is omitted.

Timing of Dosing

The importance of timing doses to achieve the maximum clinical effects has been briefly discussed above. However, patients should be instructed that NSAIDs in general do not achieve maximal effects suddenly (although see below), and that clinical response to dosing with this type of drug is unlike the pain relief from a headache - occurring within only half an hour of taking a pure analgesic.

Knowledge concerning the pharmacokinetics and pharmacodynamics of different NSAIDs varies, but aspirin and indomethacin have been studied in considerable detail, and some comments about their metabolism will emphasise the points made previously.

When used as an anti-inflammatory agent (as opposed to a simple analgesic), aspirin requires a constant ingested dose for a week before a plateau is reached (Gibson et al., 1975). Moreover, when this has been achieved, the

Table 6.2. Frequency of administration of NSAIDs[a]

Drugs	Once daily	Twice daily	Three times daily	Four or more times daily
Salicylates				
Aspirin				√
Diflunisal		√		
Benorylate		√ (suspension)	√ (tablets)	
Propionic acid derivatives				
Ibuprofen				√
Naproxen		√		
Ketoprofen				√
Fenoprofen				√
Flurbiprofen				√
Fenbufen		√		
Indole derivatives				
Indomethacin			√	
Sulindac		√		
Tolmetin				√
Phenylacetic acid derivatives				
Diclofenac			√	
Fenclofenac[b]		√		
Pyrazoles and derivatives				
Phenylbutazone[c]			√	
Oxyphenbutazone[b]			√	
Azapropazone				√
Feprazone			√	
Fenamates				
Mefenamic acid			√	
Flufenamic acid			√	
Oxicams				
Piroxicam	√			

a When a range is given the maximal frequency is shown.
b Recently withdrawn in the UK.
c Available in the UK only for treatment of ankylosing spondylitis under hospital control.

synovial fluid concentration equilibrates at a value considerably less than that of plasma. In the early stages of salicylate medication, dosing up to 6 times a day is preferable. However, after a plateau has been reached, the dosing frequency can be reduced to 4 times or even twice daily (see chapter 5, p.76).

With indomethacin, relief is usually attained within 24 hours although the maximum anti-inflammatory effect may not be obtained until a month or so of continued medication.

The timing of medication in relation to food, drink and additional medication should take into consideration several factors. In general, NSAIDs are usually given with or immediately after food but they may be better tolerated by the gastrointestinal tract if taken with antacid before food (see chapter 5, p.80); it is normal practice to encourage a reasonable fluid intake when patients are taking long term NSAID therapy, particularly if this is aspirin. Regarding salicylates, Leonards and Levy (1972) recommend the use of soluble aspirin dissolved in 15ml water, mixed with a regular dose of magnesium- or calcium-based antacid.

As most NSAIDs are potential gastric irritants it would seem reasonable to avoid mixing their ingestion with alcohol. Patients should be advised to anticipate social events so that NSAID therapy can be taken well before or well after periods of alcohol consumption. Alternatively, the occasional dose of NSAID can be omitted altogether without ill effect.

With some NSAIDs co-administration of another drug interferes with absorption (see chapter 4, p.64). One example is the reduced absorption (40%) of diflunisal by aluminum hydroxide. Another example is the reduced absorption of phenylbutazone by cholestyramine. (Although not an NSAID, it might be mentioned here that the absorption of penicillamine is inhibited by antacids, oral iron, and zinc sulfate.)

Other interactions involving NSAIDs, but not specifically their absorption, include increased plasma concentrations of indomethacin by probenecid, and the inhibition of probenecid and sulfinpyrazone by aspirin.

Reformulations: Advantages and Drawbacks

General Comment

Impressive ingenuity has been exercised in marketing new NSAIDs and, moreover, in discovering new ways to administer them.

In an era when we still have no cure for rheumatoid arthritis and many other common rheumatoses, our efforts are largely directed to symptomatic relief using drugs that are well tolerated. The newer NSAIDs are not considered to be more therapeutically effective as analgesic/anti-inflammatory agents, but many of them are less toxic and better tolerated than the classical 'yardstick' drug, aspirin. Moreover, the development of a wide range of preparations – sustained-release capsules, suspensions, suppositories, injections – even chewing gum and granules for adding to beverages – can only be regarded as an advance towards promoting *acceptability,* as well as tolerability. There is little doubt that many patients will reject a particular drug if administered in form A but accept it if in form B. For example, patients with difficulty in swallowing may prefer a suspension or the use of suppositories. On the other hand, patients offered suppositories may prefer an oral route of administration for esthetic reasons or simply because 'there is nothing wrong with my bowels'! There is also some evidence from aspirin studies that some alternatives (e.g. enteric coating, buffering, soluble forms or sodium

Table 6.3. Scope of presentations of NSAIDs [fenclofenac (Flenac) has now been withdrawn in the UK]

Tablet or capsule	Special tablet or capsule[a]	Suspension	Suppository	Injection	Other
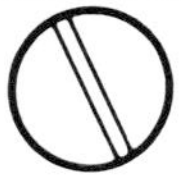	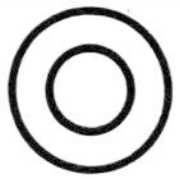	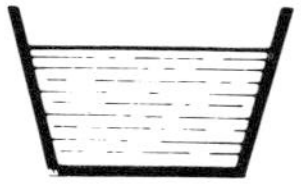	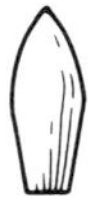	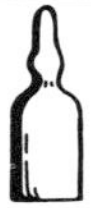	
Aspirin	Aspirin				Aspirin (chewing gum)
Diflunisal					
Benorylate		Benorylate			Benorylate (beverage granules)
Trisalicylate					
Salsalate					
Sodium salicylate		Sodium salicylate			
Ibuprofen					
Naproxen			Naproxen		
Ketoprofen			Ketoprofen		
Fenoprofen	Fenoprofen				
Flurbiprofen					
Fenbufen					
Tiaprofenic acid					
Sutoprofen					
Indomethacin	Indomethacin	Indomethacin	Indomethacin		
Sulindac					
Tolmetin					
Diclofenac	Diclofenac	Diclofenac	Diclofenac[c]	Diclofenac	
Fenclofenac[b]					
Phenylbutazone	Phenylbutazone[d]		Phenylbutazone[d]	Phenylbutazone[d]	
Azapropazone					
Feprazone[d]					
Mefenamic acid		Mefenamic acid			
Flufenamic acid					
Piroxicam					

a E.g. enteric-coated, sustained-release.
b Withdrawn in the UK.
c Pediatric suppositories also available.
d Withdrawn in the UK except for treatment of ankylosing spondylitis under hospital control.

Table 6.4. The range of NSAIDs available in the UK

Approved name	Proprietary or brand name of commercial products available in the UK
Salicylates	
Aspirin	Claradin, Laboprin, Paynocil, Caprin, Levius, Nu-Seals Aspirin, Palaprin Forte, Aspergum
Diflunisal	Dolobid
Benorylate	Benoral
Trisalicylate	Trilisate
Salsalate	Disalcid
Sodium salicylate	–
Propionic acid derivatives	
Ibuprofen	Brufen, Ebufac, Apsifen, Uniprofen
Naproxen	Naprosyn, Synflex
Ketoprofen	Orudis, Alrheumat
Fenoprofen	Fenopron, Progesic
Flurbiprofen	Froben
Fenbufen	Lederfen
Indoprofen	Flosint (suspended)
Tiaprofenic acid	Surgam
Sutoprofen	Suprol
Indole derivatives	
Indomethacin	Indocid, Imbrilon, Artracin, Indoflex, Indolar, Mobilan
Sulindac	Clinoril
Tolmetin	Tolectin
Phenylacetic acid derivatives	
Diclofenac	Voltarol
Fenclofenac[a]	Flenac (suspended)
Pyrazoles and derivatives	
Phenylbutazone[a]	Butazolidine, Butazone
Oxyphenbutazone[a]	Tanderil
Azapropazone	Rheumox
Feprazone[a]	Methrazone
Fenamates	
Mefenamic acid	Ponstan
Flufenamic acid	Meralen
Oxicams	
Piroxicam	Feldene

a Recently withdrawn in the UK (except for the use of phenylbutazone for treating ankylosing spondylitis under hospital control).

salicylate) will reduce gastrointestinal bleeding, as well as dyspepsia (Champion et al., 1975). The range of presentations of NSAIDs is summarized in table 6.3 and the commercially available products in table 6.4. The therapeutic indications are outlined in table 6.5.

Table 6.5. Therapeutic scope (based on the support of at least two clinical trials or general acclaim)

Drugs	Rheumatoid arthritis	Ankylosing spondylitis	Gout	Juvenile arthritis
Salicylates				
Aspirin	√			√
Diflunisal	√			
Benorylate	√			√
Propionic acid derivatives				
Ibuprofen	√	√		√
Naproxen	√	√	√	√
Ketoprofen	√	√		
Fenoprofen	√	√		
Flurbiprofen	√	√		
Fenbufen	√	√		
Indole derivatives				
Indomethacin	√	√	√	√
Sulindac	√	√	√	
Tolmetin	√			√
Phenylacetic acid derivatives				
Diclofenac	√			
Fenclofenac[a]	√			
Pyrazoles and derivatives				
Phenylbutazone[a]		√	√	
Oxyphenbutazone[a]		√	√	
Azapropazone	√		√	
Feprazone[a]	√			
Fenamates				
Mefenamic acid	√			
Flufenamic acid	√			
Oxicams				
Piroxicam	√	√	√	

a Recently withdrawn in the UK (except for the use of phenylbutazone for treating ankylosing spondylitis under hospital control).

The availability of drugs of different chemical character is also important as there is little doubt that the pharmacogenetic differences between patients are significant. For example, a drug of generic group A may be totally ineffective in an individual in whom a drug of generic group B is effective. The converse may be seen in another patient. Indeed this effect may even be observed within generic groups, for example, differences between the individual propionic acid derivatives.

In view of the complexity and variability of the therapeutic response to antirheumatic agents, it is useful to have several options with which to work. A couple of decades ago, of course, the only choice was between aspirin, phenylbutazone and indomethacin, and before that, aspirin alone. On the other hand, it has been argued that a constellation of drugs such as is now available prevents individual rheumatologists from gaining adequate experience of them all. There is also some evidence to suggest that newer forms of administration are no more effective than the classical oral route; for example, this has been shown with indomethacin in suppository form (Huskisson et al., 1970).

However, despite these points, the writer feels that the benefits of the availability of such a wide range of NSAID products outweighs the disadvantages.

Presentation, Packaging and Storage

Presentation

As discussed above, the scope for prescribing is increased not only by increasing the available chemical preparations but also by the variety in their presentation (table 6.3). Some specific examples will help to emphasize this:

1) Patients whose arthritis is well controlled by a particular drug may have unacceptable side effects that can be circumvented by prescribing the same drug in a different presentation. For example, patients unable to tolerate plain aspirin may be able to tolerate the soluble, buffered, enteric-coated, or micro-encapsulated preparation.

2) Patients with difficulty in swallowing tablets – particularly children and the elderly – may find the suspension form of the drug more acceptable. Alternatively, the drug can be given as a suppository.

3) Despite some evidence to the contrary, the mode of presentation may make a difference to the therapeutic response. For example, suppositories of some drugs may be more effective than the same drug taken as tablets (although, as previously stated, this has not been shown with indomethacin).

4) Patients with severely deformed hands may find a suspension presented in an easy-to-handle container (e.g. a container of benorylate with flip-off top) easier to take than tablets or suppositories. The latter, as might be expected, are particularly difficult to self-administer if hand function is severely disturbed.

5) Children may feel less inhibited taking drugs presented as an attractively colored flavored suspension. (However, the attractiveness of such preparations, and of some colored tablets, should lead to special caution in preventing accidental poisoning in children, whether patients or others.)

6) The availability of injectable forms of the drug may be invaluable in certain circumstances. For some years phenylbutazone has been available in injectable form and more recently an injectable form of diclofenac has been marketed. Injectable drugs can be of occasional use in treating acute gout, although it should be mentioned that the Committee on Safety of Medicines in the United Kingdom has now recommended that phenylbutazone be reserved for treating ankylosing spondylitis.

Packaging

The packaging as well as the presentation of drugs is important and has become more sophisticated (some might say too sophisticated) in recent years. Some of the advantages and disadvantages of modern NSAID packaging are exemplified by the following:

1) Many containers possess easily manipulable caps. These are either of the 'flip-off' type or various patterns of screw cap designed to provide an easier grip (e.g. 'wing-nut', 6-sided or 3-sided container caps).

2) Some NSAIDs are now packaged in 'pop-up' form with the intention of increasing convenience and compliance. However, patients with severely impaired hand function may find these difficult to manipulate.

3) Suppositories are a useful adjunct to rheumatic prescribing but care must be taken to explain to patients how they should be used. One pharmaceutical company has included useful illustrated instructionswith the suppository package to cover this point. However, despite earnest efforts by various means to avoid misuse, one still finds patients ingesting suppositories, inserting them nasally, or using them via the correct route but still wrapped in metal foil, or, as happened recently, in the finger stall provided for hygienic purposes.

4) Not all packaging is designed for easy use and the modern tendency to package everything in tough plastic or metal foil can lead to as much frustration for the patient as for the air passengers trying to break into a meal.

Storage

In general, medical staff and patients are insufficiently aware of correct storage instructions for NSAIDs. For example, the 'Laboprin' form of aspirin (which is hygroscopic) should be kept in a closed manufacturer's container, suppositories should be kept cool to prevent them from softening or melting and the life of diluted syrup suspensions of NSAID preparations (e.g. ibuprofen, naproxen, mefenamic acid) is only 14 days. Also, some preparations should be stored away from direct sunlight. This is stated in the manufacturer's details but may not be mentioned on the label of the bottle.

Compliance

It is an established fact that getting patients to follow medical advice is a major problem in many long term diseases, not least the rheumatic diseases. Levels of compliance are often much lower than expected and are associated with poor therapeutic effect (Capell et al., 1979; Marston, 1970; Porter, 1969).

Joyce (1962) has drawn attention to non-compliance in drug-taking in rheumatic patients. In his study, only 38 out of 108 urine samples contained the marker for the drug administered (phenylbutazone).

Other studies (Becker et al., 1972; Davis and Eichlorn, 1963; Elling, 1960; Rosenstock, 1966) have suggested a number of factors associated with compliance. These include (a) expectations and social support received by the patient from others; (b) educational attainment; and (c) socioeconomic status.

Carpenter and Davis (1976) found thatin arthritic patients, non-compliers were less likely to be housewives and were significantly more likely to be on additional drug therapy. It is not known why this should be so. They also found that instruction pamphlets, together with personal in-hospital instruction (concerning an exercise program) may be more useful than personal instruction alone. Professional home visits by remedial staff or nurses were not found to increase compliance.

Little is known about the merits of reducing the frequency of drug dosage in the hope that this will improve compliance, although one has the subjective feeling that it is helpful.

NSAIDs as Analgesics

Sometimes NSAIDs are of use in chronic arthritic conditions as analgesics 'on demand' although not all are ideal for this e.g.piroxicam when given in a single daily dose of 20 to 30mg: smaller doses appear to be ineffective and bigger doses no more effective but less well tolerated by the gastrointestinal tract. Moreover, the drug takes several days to reach steady-state and thus its peak of anti-inflammatory efficacy is delayed.

Some NSAIDs are used as analgesics in non-rheumatic disorders (e.g. dysmenorrhea in which inhibition of cyclo-oxygenase appears to be a feature), and extension of this to rheumatic disorders has some attraction for patients with rheumatic diseases that run a variable course and requireintermittent rather than continuous dosage.

NSAIDs found to be useful as analgesics include the classical one – aspirin – as well as fenoprofen, ibuprofen, naproxen,naproxen sodium, diflunisal (Hart and Huskisson, 1984), ketoprofen, flurbiprofen, mefenamic acid, indomethacin and proquazone. When the choice between an NSAID and a plain analgesic [e.g. acetaminophen, propoxyphene (dextropropoxyphene)] arises, the NSAID has the merit of an additional anti-inflammatory action and possibly increased safety in overdosage. The traditional analgesic, on the other hand, is cheaper.

NSAIDs in Clinical Perspective

The rapid proliferation of NSAIDs, their similar efficacy and apparent inability to significantly alter fundamental disease processes, may give rise to the view that we have sufficient drugs of this class.

When aspirin was the bedrock of NSAID therapy, clinicians could explore alternative approaches only within the confines of that drug: for instance, trying soluble, enteric-coated and other formulations, and attempting to modify therapeutic effects and toxicity by subtle manipulation of dosage, timing, and the effects of co-administration of alkalis. With the advent of the NSAIDs this detailed approach seems to have been replaced by a natural temptation to reach for an alternative drug, perhaps without giving the first a fair trial. Put another way, has the philosophy of therapeutic *management* been replaced by one of *treatment,* the latter term being used in a more restrictive sense than the former?

At present, of necessity, drug use in rheumatology involves a blend of analgesics, analgesic-anti-inflammatories (NSAIDs), corticosteroids and, in rheumatoid arthritis, remittive agents. A welcome advance would be the replacement of this polypharmacy with a single drug. This may be impossible, but a hint of what could lie ahead may rest in the suspicion that three NSAIDs, alclofenac, fenclofenac and benoxaprofen, may influence the basic disease process as well as the symptoms of pain and inflammation. Because all three have been withdrawn from general use (at least temporarily) this remains but a hint. However, work with fenclofenac has been allowed to continue (Berry et al., 1980) and we await the results with interest.

References

Australasian Multicentre Trial Group: The simultaneous assessment of four non-steroidal anti-inflammatory drugs in rheumatoid arthritis using a simple and rapid trial design. Journal of Rheumatology 7: 857-864 (1980).

Baum, J.: Ethical aspects of drug therapy in children. Clinical Rheumatology 1: 45-46 (1982).

Becker, M.H.; Drachman, R.H. and Kirscht, J.P.: Predicting mothers' compliance with pediatric regimes. Journal of Pediatrics 81: 843-854 (1972).

Berry, H.; Ford-Hutchinson, A.W.; Camp, A.V.; Heywood, D.; Molloy, M.G.; James, D.W. and Hamilton, E.B.D.: Antirheumatic activity of alclofenac. Annals of the Rheumatic Diseases 39: 473-475 (1980).

Bibace, R. and Walsh, M.E.: Development of children's concepts of illness. Pediatrics 66: 912-917 (1980).

Capell, H.A.; Rennie, J.A.N. and Rooney, P.J.: Patient compliance: A novel method of testing non-steroidal anti-inflammatory analgesics in rheumatoid arthritis. Journal of Rheumatology 6: 584-593 (1979).

Carpenter, J.O. and Davis, L.J.: Medical recommendations – followed or ignored? Factors influencing compliance in arthritis. Archives of Physical Medicine and Rehabilitation 57: 241-246 (1976).

Champion, C.D.; Day, R.O.; Graham, G.G. and Paull, P.D.: Salicylates in rheumatoid arthritis; in Pearson and Dick (Eds) Clinics in the Rheumatic Diseases, pp.245-265 (Saunders, London 1975).

Davis, M.S. and Eichlorn, R.L.: Compliance with medical regimens: Panel study. Journal of Health and Human Behaviour 4: 240 (1963).

Gall, E.P.; Capeerton, E.M.; McComb, J.E.; Nessmer, R.; Multz, C.V.; O'Hanlan, M. and Willkens, R.F.: Clinical comparison of ibuprofen, fenoprofen, calcium, naproxen and tolmetin sodium in rheumatoid arthritis. Journal of Rheumatology 9: 402-407 (1982).Elling, R.; Whittemore, R. and Green, M.: Patient participation in a pediatric program. Journal of Health and Human Behaviour 1: 183 (1960).

Gibson, T.; Zaphiropoulos, G.; Grove, J.; Widdop, B. and Barry, D.: Kinetics of salicylate metabolism. British Journal of Clinical Pharmacology 2: 233-238 (1975).

Hart, F.D. and Huskisson, E.C.: Non-steroidal anti-inflammatory drugs. Current status and rational therapeutic use. Drugs 27: 232-255 (1984).

Huskisson, E.C.; Taylor, R.T.; Burston, D.; Chuter, P.J. and Hart, F.D.: Evening indomethacin in the treatment of rheumatoid arthritis. Annals of the Rheumatic Diseases 28: 393-396 (1970).

Huskisson, E.C.; Woolf, D.L.; Balme, H.W.; Scott, J. and Franklyn, S.: Four new anti-inflammatory drugs: Responses and variations. British Medical Journal 1: 1048-1050 (1976).

Joyce, C.R.B.: Patient cooperation and the sensitivity of clinical trials. Journal of Chronic Diseases 15: 1025 (1962).

Laurence, D.R.: Clinical Pharmacology, 4th ed., p.19 (Churchill Livingstone, Edinburgh 1973).

Leonards, J.R. and Levy, G.: Effect of pharmaceutical formulation on gastrointestinal bleeding from aspirin tablets. Archives of Internal Medicine 129: 457-460 (1972).

Marston, M.V.: Compliance with medical regimens: Review of literature. Nursing Research 19: 312-323 (1970).

Porter, A.M.: Drug defaulting in general practice. British Medical Journal 1: 218 (1969).

Reynolds, P.M.G. and Whorwell, P.J.: A single blind crossover comparison of fenoprofen, ibuprofen and naproxen in rheumatoid arthritis. Current Medical Research and Opinion 2: 461-463 (1974).
Rosenstock, I.M.: Why people use health services. Milbank Memorial Fund Quarterly 44: 94 (1966).
Wasner, C.; Button, M.C.; Kraines, R.G.; Kaye, R.L.; Bobrove, A.M. and Fries, J.F.: Non-steroidal anti-inflammatory agents in rheumatoid arthritis and ankylosing spondylitis. Journal of the American Medical Association 246: 2168-2172 (1981).

Further Reading

Bird, H.A. and Wright, V.: Applied Drug Therapy of the Rheumatic Diseases (Wright PSG, Bristol 1982).
Hart, F.D. (Ed.): Drug Treatment of the Rheumatic Diseases, 2nd ed. (ADIS Health Science Press, Sydney 1982).
Hart, F.D. and Huskisson, E.C.: Non-steroidal anti-inflammatory drugs. Current status and rational therapeutic use. Drugs 27: 232-255 (1984).
Moll, J.M.H.: Management of Rheumatic Disorders (Chapman and Hall, London 1983).
Moll, J.M.H.; Bird, H.A. and Rushton, A. (Eds): Therapeutics in Rheumatology (Chapman and Hall, London. In press 1985).
Verbeeck, R.K.; Blackburn, J.L. and Loewen, G.R.: Clinical pharmacokinetics of non-steroidal anti-inflammatory drugs. Clinical Pharmacokinetics 8: 297-331 (1983).

7. Choosing and Prescribing NSAIDs

F. Dudley Hart

London, England

While the importance of diagnosing the arthritic condition correctly is universally accepted today, it was not so apparent to our forbears who, while accepting the importance of diagnosing cardiac, pulmonary and abdominal conditions correctly, were rather less strict in the arthritic disorders. Largely, this was because even as recently as 50 years ago the rheumatic diseases were lumped together into a handful of conditions which were imperfectly studied and poorly defined. As a student, I can remember my chiefs saying, 'In medicine, there is diagnosis, prognosis and occasionally effective therapy'. This is true, perhaps, of much of rheumatology today. Diagnostic criteria have been refined but still need further refinement.

Importance of Correct Diagnosis and Severity of Disease

Osteoarthritis

Osteoarthritis is no longer a diagnosis of one disease, but of a group of conditions with varying clinical and pathological manifestations. The same may prove in the future to be true of rheumatoid arthritis. In southern England, a large house-to-house survey of the rheumatic disorders several years ago had to be abandoned as the first investigator in the field had not distinguished generalized osteoarthritis from rheumatoid arthritis; while this would seem unlikely to occur today, these two conditions can still be and are confused, and polymyalgia rheumatica is frequently misdiagnosed as rheumatoid arthritis or vice versa. As patients with polymyalgia rheumatica are usually elderly and frequently have osteoarthritic changes this may also cause diagnostic confusion. Not infrequently elderly patients with radiological evidence of degenerative disease are thought to be suffering from osteoarthritis when their symptoms are unrelated to the disease and in many cases are due to anxiety or tension states, depression, boredom or unhappiness. In such cases, anxiolytic or antidepressive agents are much more likely to produce relief of symptoms than are analgesics or non-steroidal anti-inflammatory agents. Radiological changes are not necessarily related to symptoms, as was nicely illustrated by a study reported last year in a London hospital (Heller et al., 1983). In one year, 85% of patients aged 60 or more referred for an examination of the neck were reported as having cervical spondylosis. Much the same figure was obtained in a control series of patients who attended for barium studies and who had no complaints relating to the neck. There was no significant difference in the prevalence of radiological evidence of cervical spondylosis between the two groups. Though the severity of disc changes was greater among the complainers than the controls, there was no consistent relationship between symptoms and radiological changes.

Rheumatoid Arthritis

In the management of a chronic painful condition it is important to take into account the emotional factors which prevail with prolonged suffering and to assess, as best one can, what particular factors are operating in the patient under consideration. In rheumatoid arthritis (Hart, 1980, 1982) the 'pain-mix' is a cocktail of discomforts arising from systemic 'illness', local joint and ligamentous pains, joint swelling, muscle weakness and stiffness, anxiety, depression, effects of the therapy being given, boredom, feelings of being thwarted and sometimes extra-articular manifestations such as neuropathy, pericarditis or vasculitis. Resentment adds to and intensifies this diabolical cocktail.

In osteoarthritis, the overtones are fewer and systemic illness arising from the arthritis is nil or slight. However, other considerations enter the picture, for a patient in this older age group tends to have other disorders for which he or she may be receiving treatment so that polypharmacy is more common and drug reactions and interactions more frequent. Elderly patients do not handle drugs as well as younger subjects and are often receiving several drugs for several disorders.

Rheumatoid arthritis and osteoarthritis may affect one, a few or several joints mildly, moderately or severely, and a considerable amount of literature has been published in an attempt to give measurable values to the different components present in a given patient. Many years ago, Lansbury, (1958) described his articular and systemic indices for rheumatoid arthritis which were used in clinical trials in the assessment of new corticosteroids and NSAIDs, preceding and making the way for the simpler Ritchie Articular Index which has now been in general use in antirheumatic drug trials for many years (Ritchie et al., 1968). Mason et al. (1967) and many other workers since have devised schemes for measuring clinical parameters which could allow for the variability of joint involvement and systemic upset, one of the latest being the multivariate analysis in assessment of disease activity in rheumatoid arthritis by Mallya and Mace (1981). This comprises morning stiffness, pain scale, grip strength, articular index, hemoglobin and erythrocyte sedimentation rate. Doyle et al. (1981) have produced a modified articular index for use in osteoarthritic studies. An entire issue of Clinics in Rheumatic Diseases has recently been devoted to clinical trials in the rheumatic diseases, with a chapter on rheumatoid arthritis and NSAIDs by Paulus (1983) and degenerative joint disease by Altman and Hochberg (1983).

Gout

Gout, though extremely painful during an acute attack, is not usually accompanied by systemic or psychiatric illness and is an agonising event, not a chronic painful, soul-destroying disorder. For this reason it is easier to treat. Indeed, the ability to rapidly control such an acute attack is a fair measure of anti-inflammatory potency of an NSAID; although pains may be severe the NSAIDs usually rapidly bring relief and have replaced colchicine and the corticosteroids in the treatment of acute attacks.

Interpatient Variation

It has to be re-emphasised that all the chronic arthropathies vary greatly in severity, extent and duration, so much so that it has been said in the past that no two groups of patients with rheumatoid arthritis are truly alike, even in the most carefully organized clinical trials, whether paired for age, sex, disease duration and other factors, and that comparing two forms of therapy in apparently similar groups may give results which depend as much on the underlying disease as the treatment given (see also chapter 2). This is partly true, but with the NSAIDs we are not expecting complete resolution but symptomatic improvement and such improvement can be measured in different ways.

According to Bombadier et al. (1982) speaking in Canada on the outcomes in rheumatological clinical trials, there was general agreement that in rheumatoid arthritis the most useful measurements were joint count, pain score, global assessment, morning stiffness and grip strength, though these measurements were not truly independent of each other. Vallance (1982) in a review of clinical trials noted that most clinical trials comparing the efficacy of two NSAIDs failed to show any difference between them, the conclusion often being drawn that the two were equally effective. But he points out that half of such trials had an unacceptable probability of missing a real difference of 25% between treatments, and 80% of studies could have missed a 15% difference, though most of the studies could have detected a 50% difference between treatments if such had been present. He notes that to conclude that two treatments are equal, based on a statistical finding of no significant difference, is not justified unless the probability of the β-error is reported – the β-error calculations determining the probability of missing a true difference between treatments when no significant difference has been found.

Spontaneous Remission

Another factor which should be considered is spontaneous remission of the disease. Professor Klinenberg (see chapter 1) points out that natural remission is common in the first year of rheumatoid arthritis. This may bedevil assessments of drug efficacy and it was for this reason that the European Rheumatism Council's Gold Trial (1960) included only patients who had had the disease for 1 to 5 years. The ability of a drug to induce remission is all

Table 7.1. Criteria for clinical remission in rheumatoid arthritis[a]

Five or more of the following requirements must be fulfilled for at least 2 consecutive months:
1. Duration of morning stiffness not exceeding 15 minutes
2. No fatigue
3. No joint pain (by history)
4. No joint tenderness or pain on motion
5. No soft tissue swelling in joints or tendon sheaths
6. ESR (Westergren method) < 30mm/h (female) or 20mm/h (male)

a From Primer on Rheumatic Diseases, 8th ed., p.208 (Arthritis Foundation, Atlanta 1983).

important but difficult to assess. For this reason a list of proposed criteria for clinical remission has been devised (table 7.1).

In the 1940s, Short and Bauer (1948) studied a group of 250 patients receiving only simple medical treatment. Almost 10% of them were in clinical remission for 12 to 31 years (mean 22 years) but it is worth noting that when enrolled for the study most patients had had their disease for less than 6 months.

One never knows which patients with rheumatoid arthritis will go into remission. In general, those with acute onset of disease are more likely to do so, while remission is much less likely in patients with strongly seropositive disease with nodules. The future effective therapy of rheumatoid arthritis may well lie particularly in this field. Meanwhile which agent is most likely to switch off this unpleasant disease? Unfortunately there is no good evidence that any NSAID does so.

Presence of Complicating Disease and Need for Other Drug Treatment

Osteoarthritic patients are often elderly and not infrequently have other disorders which need to be treated. Polypharmacy is therefore required in many elderly patients and side effects and interaction of drugs are more common.

In arthritic patients the more common coexisting disorders which might need treatment with other drugs are peptic ulcers, hiatus herniae, ischemic and/or hypertensive heart disease, chronic bronchitis, asthma and skin disorders. It is as well before starting NSAID therapy to enquire also about the patient's tobacco and alcohol consumption. Any NSAID may cause dyspepsia or gastrointestinal upsets, edema of the extremities and some diminution in renal function from prostaglandin inhibition but dyspepsia is the most common. Skin reactions of various kinds are less common but have contributed or led to the withdrawal of certain agents in the past, e.g. alclofenac and benoxaprofen. Patients who have had allergic reactions to aspirin may develop them with other NSAIDs (D'Arcy, 1983; Rake and Jacobs, 1983).

Drug-Induced Edema

It was noted with phenylbutazone in the early days of its use in the chronic arthropathies that edema might be induced, and in a study by Smyth and Percy (1973) it was noted that though pain was relieved by phenylbutazone as it was by indomethacin in acute gout, swelling was reduced with the latter but not with the former drug. More recently edema of the feet was a frequent finding in patients treated with piroxicam in a geriatric unit (Fowler and Arnold, 1983). Athough Nuki (1983) in a review of the NSAIDs states that piroxicam appears to be a safe form of drug therapy in the elderly which does not accumulate in patients with renal impairment despite its long half-life (see chapter 5, table 5.1), Fowler and Arnold (1983) point out that in their geriatric unit in London, they have seen 6 patients in heart failure which they considered due to this drug; in 3 there was a clear relationship to piroxicam administration. They consider that piroxicam can precipitate severe congestive heart failure and that it is overprescribed in the elderly and should not be used as a first-line drug. It is fair to point out, however, that cardiac failure occurred some weeks after piroxicam had been started and that 2 patients were also taking tin and tin oxide tablets ('Stanoxyl') which are likely to have the same effect.

Yeung Laiwah and Mactier (1981) and others have drawn attention to the antagonistic effect of the NSAIDs on furosemide-induced diuresis in cardiac failure. Edema of the feet and ankles may be seen on occasions with most, if not all, of the NSAIDs, though in the geriatric population it is difficult, if not impossible, to know how much of this peripheral edema is due to the NSAID or to immobility and disuse, cardiac and/or renal disease, low plasma proteins or poor venous return. Frequently several of these factors operate and edema around an inflamed ankle or foot in a patient with rheumatoid arthritis can be due to involvement of those joints by this disease.

Drug Interactions

The drugs most often given in the elderly population are diuretics and digitalis, antihypertensive drugs of different types, laxatives and anticoagulants for thromboembolic, vascular and cardiovascular disorders. These complicate therapy as there are predictable clinically significant interactions between the coumarin anticoagulants and phenylbutazone and oxyphenbutazone.

Diuretics may increase plasma uric acid levels and precipitate acute attacks of gout and, rarely, tophus formation. Some NSAIDs given with anticoagulant therapy may cause hemorrhage in a joint or elsewhere (chapter 4, p.64). Phenylbutazone is contraindicated in the presence of renal and hepatic disease, including recent hepatitis. It may also potentiate certain antidiabetic oral hypoglycemic agents and sulfonamides, necessitating a reduction of dosage.

Introduced in 1952, phenylbutazone was the first of the non-steroidal anti-inflammatory agents since aspirin was marketed at the turn of the century. Phenylbutazone retained its place in therapeutics until this year, when, apart from its use for ankylosing spondylitis, under hospital control at hospitals in Great Britain, it has been withdrawn from the market since a number of other effective, less toxic NSAIDs are now available. It is certainly true that cross-reactions with other drugs, though seldom serious, are more common with aspirin and phenylbutazone than with their successors though it is also true that they have been in general use over much longer periods than their successors (chapter 4, table 4.1).

Gastrointestinal Complaints

The most common side effects with any of the NSAIDs, more so with some than with others, are nausea, dyspepsia and gastrointestinal irritation – a partly local effect on the gastric mucosa, partly via the blood, but mostly

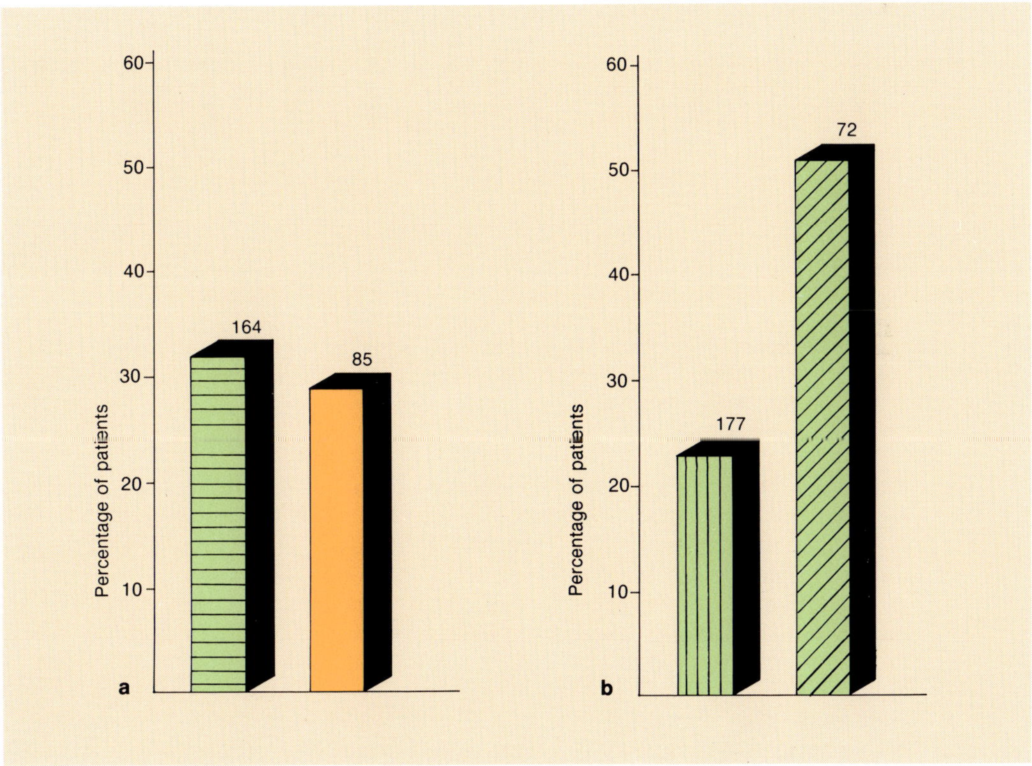

Fig. 7.1.
(**a**) Incidence of endoscopically verified gastric lesions in patients with rheumatoid arthritis ▤ or osteoarthritis ▢ after at least 3 months' treatment with NSAIDs (189) or a corticosteroid (60).
(**b**) Incidence of gastric lesions in patients with rheumatoid arthritis or osteoarthritis treated with a single drug ▥ or combined drug therapy ▨ (after Caruso and Bianchi Porro, 1980a).

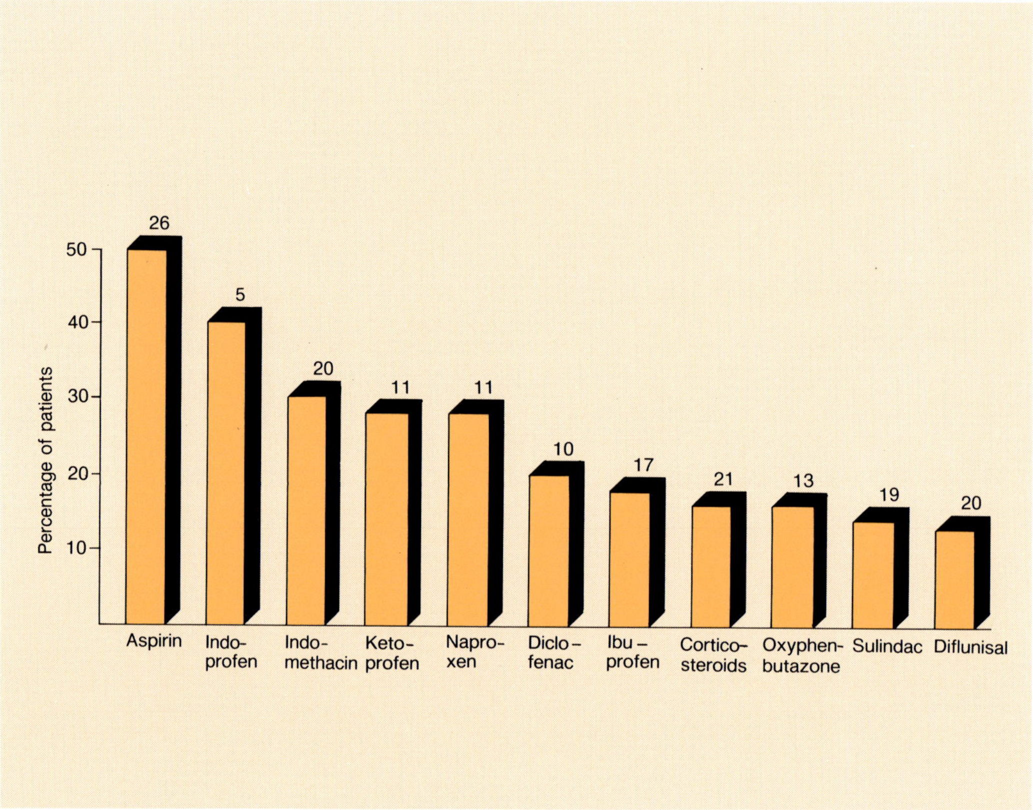

Fig. 7.2. Incidence of endoscopically verified gastric lesions after at least 3 months' treatment with a single NSAID or a corticosteroid in patients with rheumatoid arthritis or osteoarthritis (after Caruso and Bianchi Porro, 1980a). Number above columns represents patients who received each drug.

the former. Normally a mucous gel layer protects the gastric mucosa, trapping bicarbonate. Prostaglandins stimulate and enhance this effect and also aid in mucosal repair after injury. The NSAIDs, however, are mucolytic and negate the prostaglandin protective effect, leading to cell death.

Caruso and Bianchi Porro (1980a,b) in a gastroscopic study of 164 rheumatoid patients and 85 osteoarthritics treated with NSAIDs or corticosteroids for several months found that gastric lesions occurred with similar frequency in both types of disease but were more frequent in patients who were treated with more than one drug (fig. 7.1). Gastric ulcer was defined as a sharply circumscribed 3-dimensional lesion with a white base (Silvoso et al., 1979), gastric erosions as superficial white 2-dimensional defects in the gastric mucosa, mild mucosal erythema and/or hyperemia being ignored and classed as normal.

Aspirin, as found in other studies (see chapter 3), proved more irritant to the gastric mucosa than other drugs studied (fig. 7.2.). There was a lack of correlation between the patients' symptoms and the gastroscopic findings, 17 of 41 (41%) patients having gastroscopic lesions with no complaints, 28 of 136 (21%) having complaints but no gastroscopic abnormality.

In the correspondence following this paper, the potential hazards of gastroscopy with diazepam sedation in rheumatoid patients with atlanto-axial subluxation was raised (Oldham, 1980).

Influence of Alcohol and Tobacco

It is worth noting that in very few studies of gastric complications with NSAIDs is there any mention of other drugs being given concurrently or of cigarette smoking habits or alcohol consumption. Such figures might be found to be different in non-smokers and smokers and it is known that heavy alcohol consumption in patients on aspirin and probably also on other NSAIDs is likely to precipitate gastric bleeding.

Alcohol and tobacco consumption may affect side effects of drugs and in themselves produce side effects which may be misinterpreted. Cigarette smoke contains a large number of chemicals, the most important from the point of view of effects on drug activity being polycyclic aromatic hydrocarbons as they are powerful hepatic microsomal enzyme inducers. Enzyme induction can cause adverse reactions by altering the steady-state concentrations of drugs administered long term, particularly those cleared by hepatic metabolism, and while this may apply more to phenothiazines, anticoagulants, antihypertensives and hypoglycemic agents than to NSAIDs, the smoking habits of patients should be noted, particularly if they are taking several drugs (Luczynska and Wilson, 1983).

In a recent study Willoughby and Essigman (unpublished) found a significant association with smoking and peptic ulcer in rheumatoid sufferers, an increase of 10 cigarettes a day being related to an increase of about 14% of peptic ulceration.

Avoiding the Problems by Drug Selection

In choosing a NSAID the patient's history may give a lead as to which NSAID to avoid, simple pharmacopoeal ('ordinary') aspirin and indomethacin being more likely to cause gastric irritation, for instance, than others. Blood loss in the stools is less with all NSAIDs than with 'ordinary' aspirin.

Now that oxyphenbutazone has been withdrawn and phenylbutazone confined to hospital treatment of ankylosing spondylitis in Great Britain, indomethacin, introduced in 1964, is the senior member of the team. It holds its place as a very effective agent with a greater tendency to cause gastrointestinal toxicity than most of the other NSAIDs; the unpleasant headaches and cerebral sensations are dose-related and lessen and disappear with dose reduction. Gastric irritation is less using the indomethacin suppository than the oral preparation (Hart and Huskisson, 1984; Whitehouse and Hart, 1965).

Ibuprofen, introduced at low dosage in Great Britian around 1969 has proved in general well tolerated and the recommended dosage has been increased, as has naproxen (see chapter 3, p.45) which was found by Huskisson et al. (1976) and Reynolds and Whorwell (1974) to be more effective than the other propionics assessed (ibuprofen, ketoprofen and fenoprofen) with fenoprofen being second in popularity. Gall et al. (1982) found in patients' and physicians' ratings, that the preference was for naproxen, ibuprofen, fenoprofen, tolmetin and aspirin in that order, though in a 10-center Australasian group trial no significant difference was found in 400 rheumatoid arthritis patients between naproxen, sulindac, salicylates and ibuprofen though all were significantly better than placebo (Australian Multicentre Trial Group, 1980). Once again Vallance's (1982) point is probably relevant; differences of less than 50% frequently fail to show in such trials comparing 2 not very dissimilar antirheumatic agents (see p.106).

Interaction of NSAIDs and oral antidiabetic drugs has been referred to in chapter 4. Salicylates, in large dosages, have been reported to enhance the hypoglycemic response to sulfonylureas. As a result caution is needed if moderate to large doses are required in patients receiving sulfonylurea hypoglycemic agents.

Similarly prolonged hypoglycemia has been reported when phenylbutazone was given to such patients. Both phenylbutazone and oxyphenbutazone inhibit carboxylation of tolbutamide, giving rise to increased serum levels, as well as displacing it from plasma protein sites. On the other hand studies with oral antidiabetic agents and diflunisal, sulindac, tolmetin, diclofenac and naproxen have not shown any significant clinical interaction though caution is advised and the close observation of patients on oral antidiabetic agents given any NSAIDs.

Considerations of Extremes of Age and Frequency of Dosage

All medical students are taught to reduce the dosage of drugs in children according to their age and bodyweight and to use only those drugs which are suitable for, and well tolerated by, children. Textbooks of applied pharmacology and therapeutics have always emphasized the importance of observing these rules in treating young patients but not until relatively recently has the same precept been observed in treating elderly patients. There are great interindividual differences in drug tolerance in the elderly. Many elderly patients show deterioration of body systems, metabolic deficiencies and suffer from several disorders with the result that adverse drug reactions occur more frequently in this group of patients than in younger subjects.

Polypharmacy

Multiple disorders often mean that several clinicians are prescribing different drugs and geriatric patients may sometimes be receiving 3 or 4 groups of drugs from 3 or 4 different specialists. In addition some drugs may be purchased over the counter, e.g. analgesics and laxatives.

The elderly tend to forget to take their medicines or forget they have, in fact, taken them and take them again, so that under- and overdosage is not unusual in the age group over 65 years, when osteoarthritis, giant cell arteritis and polymyalgia rheumatica are not uncommon and gout and rheumatoid arthritis have still to be considered in differential diagnosis.

It is extraordinary how many elderly patients do not know what their various medicines are, or what are the likely therapeutic benefits or possible side effects. Infrequent dosage once or twice a day has the great advantage of removing the need for midday and afternoon doses, which are so often forgotten, and simplifying the therapeutic regimen. A possible disadvantage of a drug with a prolonged duration of action is the production of toxic reactions from overdosage if the drug is not metabolised or eliminated normally; this is not uncommon in the elderly where hepatic and renal function may be impaired.

Impaired Liver Function

Metabolism by the liver is the main route of elimination of many drugs but the hepatic reserve is large and liver disease has to be severe before significant changes in drug metabolism occur. Routine liver function tests are of little help in general for they are a poor guide to the capacity of the liver to metabolize drugs and one can never be sure how a given drug will be dealt with by the liver of a particular patient.

Hypoproteinemia (hypoalbuminemia) in severe liver disease is associated with increased toxicity of some higher protein-bound drugs and the NSAIDs and the corticosteroids are, in general, highly protein-bound. A prolonged prothrombin time due to liver disease may affect blood clotting and predispose to hemorrhage particularly when drugs that alter platelet function are given. Edema and ascites in chronic liver disease may be accentuated by some NSAIDs and though phenylbutazone was found to act in this way several other NSAIDs may act similarly on occasion and are more likely in the presence of renal disease to cause not only fluid retention but also gastrointestinal bleeding.

Impaired Renal Function

A very real hazard is renal impairment in the elderly. Failure to excrete a drug or its metabolites may produce toxic reactions and, even if elimination is normal, toxic and hypersensitivity reactions are generally more common with drugs in the presence of renal impairment and some therapeutic agents cease to be effective. Renal impairment is arbitrarily divided into 3 grades; mild with a glomerular filtration rate (GFR) of 20 to 50 ml/min and a serum creatinine of 150 to 300 μmol/L; moderate with a GFR of 10 to 20 ml/min and a serum creatinine of 300 to 700 μmol/L; and severe when the GFR is less than 10 ml/min and serum creatinine more than 700 μmol/L. Renal function declines with age and many elderly patients have a glomerular filtration

Table 7.2. Renal kinetics of some commonly used NSAIDs

Drug	Total renal excretion (% of dose)	Unchanged drug (% of dose)	Active metabolites
Aspirin	Dose dependent	< 2	Yes
Azapropazone	≈ 90	62 (51-73)	
Diclofenac	?	< 1	
Diflunisal	80-95	< 3	
Fenbufen	65	4	Yes (unchanged drug is inactive)
Fenoprofen	96	2-5	
Indomethacin	?	< 15	
Ibuprofen	?	1	
Mefenamic acid	52	< 6	
Naproxen	> 90	< 10	
Piroxicam	?	2-5	
Sulindac	?	7	Yes (unchanged drug is inactive)
Tolmetin	≈ 90	15	

rate less than 50 ml/min which may not be reflected in changes in serum creatinine which should be corrected for age, sex and weight by nomograms.

As advised in the British National Formulary (1984) it is probably wise to assume at least a mild impairment in the elderly and prescribe somewhat smaller doses of NSAIDs and if renal impairment is severe to avoid them altogether. With NSAIDs such as azapropazone, sulindac or diflunisal, which are excreted largely by the kidney, the Formulary advises the first two not be given if the GFR is under 20 ml/min nor diflunisal if the GFR is below 10 ml/min.

Renal excretion of unchanged drug is usually small (table 7.2), the elimination of most NSAIDs depending largely on hepatic biotransformation (see chapter 5, p.72). The most notable exception is azapropazone, around 62% of which is excreted unchanged in the urine, about 20% of the dose as the 6-hydroxy derivative (Verbeeck et al., 1983).

NSAIDs in Children

In childhood, the only NSAIDs recommended by the manufacturers are aspirin, benorylate suspension, ibuprofen syrup, tolmetin and mefenamic acid, the dosage being scaled down according to age and in the case of mefenamic acid given for not more than one week. Ansell (1982), however, adds indomethacin, naproxen, diclofenac sodium and piroxicam to this list as permissible in the treatment of juvenile chronic arthritis.

NSAIDs in Pregnancy

Although there is little or no evidence that any NSAIDs have any particular adverse effect in pregnancy on mother or fetus, since the complications of treatment with thalidomide, physicians and their pregnant patients have preferred to avoid the use of NSAIDs or any other drugs in pregnancy, particularly in the first 3 months. Prostaglandin synthetase inhibitors prolong gestation in laboratory animals, and indomethacin has been used successfully to inhibit premature labor, but such drugs may produce premature closure of the ductus arteriosus when administered near term. However, there is little in the way of hard evidence in animal work or in obstetrics that the NSAIDs have in general any effect on fetal development when given to pregnant women earlier in pregnancy. Similarly, although the NSAIDs may be present in breast milk the amount is usually small though mothers wishing to breastfeed their babies are usually advised to avoid regular medication with NSAIDs.

Balancing Benefit and Risk with NSAIDs

Toxicity

As a group, the toxicity of NSAIDs compares favorably with the slow-acting agents such as gold salts or penicillamine, for the risks of blood dyscrasias and skin reactions are considerably greater in the latter. Even with certain NSAIDs carrying a risk of serious hematological and dermatological side effects (e.g. phenylbutazone and oxyphenbutazone) [see chapter 3, p.48], the risk was worth taking as such side effects were rare and clinical benefits outweighed them when there were few other NSAIDs available.

Such is not now the case and as a result these two agents have been withdrawn from general practice in the United Kingdom. Other NSAIDs withdrawn in the United Kingdom because of toxic side effects have been ibufenac (liver), alclofenac (skin), indoprofen (gastrointestinal), zomepirac (allergic), feprazone (gastrointestinal and skin) and benoxaprofen (liver, kidney and skin) and recently fenclofenac (skin). With each drug the dividing line between what is an acceptable risk and what is not depends on the drug's popularity in general practice and its effectiveness, though much publicity, as in the case of benoxaprofen, may complicate the issue, the public becoming more aware of the side effects of the drug from the media.

In general the propionic acid derivatives as a group have held their place in therapeutics well with an entirely acceptable balance between effectiveness and adverse reactions. Ibuprofen, the first of this class, was introduced at the low dosage of 200mg 3 or 4 times a day; at this dose level side effects were minimal but so were the therapeutic effects and on increasing the daily dosage to 1.8 to 2.4g, therapeutic effects were considerably more impressive while the incidence of side effects remained acceptable. Naproxen also has had its recommended dosage increased from

250mg twice daily to double this dosage, with greater therapeutic effect and good tolerance. Indomethacin, introduced around 1964, has proved an excellent and effective NSAID at the expense of not infrequent gastrointestinal upsets and headaches, dizziness and lightheadedness which occur at higher dosage but which disappear or lessen on dose reduction. Dyspepsia with this drug is not dose-related however, and occurs at almost any dosage level in some patients but not at all in others. Sulindac, an indene derivative of indomethacin, though less potent is better tolerated.

The fenamates, flufenamic and mefenamic acids, cause diarrhea in around 10% of patients, a disadvantage in most patients but a virtue in a costive minority. As Verbeeck et al. (1983) conclude in their review of the NSAIDs, in clinical practice there appear to be no clearcut guidelines to help the physician in the selection of the most appropriate one for a particular patient.

Interpatient Variability

The once- or twice-a-day dosage schedules are more popular than more frequent administration and piroxicam, diflunisal, naproxen, fenbufen and sulindac all have this advantage. Other agents, e.g. azapropazone, can also be given in an increased dosage twice a day with the same therapeutic effect as more frequent administration and diclofenac, ketoprofen and indomethacin can be administered in sustained-release form once a day.

Certain patients fail to respond to some NSAIDs while responding satisfactorily to others. Although this is often due to the balance between relief of symptoms and subclinical or mild side effects such as mild nausea or headaches, or to the taste or color of, or faith in, a certain preparation, there is evidence that some patients do respond to certain NSAIDs and fail to benefit from others apparently as a result of a different pharmacological 'handling' of the drug by the 'non-responders' (Baber et al., 1979; Orme et al., 1981). There is a greater interpatient than inter-drug variability in response and in adverse reactions.

A trial and error empirical approach is usually necessary after taking note of clinical response to previous drugs and a careful history of drug reactions and of gastrointestinal, renal, hepatic and other complaints and of allergies of all sorts, particularly to aspirin and to other NSAIDs. It is as well also to enquire about the results of previous investigations, particularly gastrointestinal. As the NSAIDs are essentially rapidly acting symptom-controlling rather than curative drugs, if no beneficial therapeutic response whatsoever is seen after 2 to 3 weeks on a given NSAID there is usually little point in persevering with it. It is quite likely that over long periods a disease-suppressing effect may occur, the disease gradually subsiding under cover of the drug, but induction of remission has not been proven so far with NSAIDs in clinical or radiological studies. Such claims have been made for immunoregulatory and long term drugs such as gold salts, D-penicillamine, azathioprine and cyclophosphamide, but the evidence in the main is inadequate: rheumatoid arthritis and other inflammatory arthropathies do spontaneously remit and symptoms wax and wane in osteoarthritis sometimes for no particular or therapeutic reason.

What is certain is that, in general, the NSAIDs are considerably less toxic and less dangerous than the long term and immunoregulatory agents, that in acute inflammatory conditions like gout they are the drugs of first choice, that in chronic or relapsing inflammatory arthropathies such as rheumatoid arthritis and the seronegative arthropathies they are first-line orthodox treatment and that in many cases of osteoarthritis they often reduce symptoms very considerably, particularly when given for inflammatory or traumatic exacerbations. If they do not produce definite symptomatic improvement there is little virtue in continuing therapy indefinitely or over long periods in osteoarthritis.

Selecting the Best NSAID

The following are some general guidelines for selection of NSAIDs for particular types of patients:

1) If an NSAID is needed largely for analgesic effect in an elderly subject with osteoarthritis or mild rheumatoid arthritis fenbufen, naproxen or ibuprofen are usually well tolerated. The first two can be given twice daily or once in the morning.

Piroxicam has the advantage of once-daily administration as has isoxicam, which is still under trial.

2) In more acute inflammatory disease, indomethacin, flurbiprofen, naproxen, diclofenac, azapropazone and fenoprofen all have an effective anti-inflammatory and analgesic action. In the treatment of acute gout, for instance, all have proved effective.

3) Where local gastric irritation limits the use of oral preparations suppositories are available in Great Britain of indomethacin (100mg), naproxen (500mg), ketoprofen (100mg), piroxicam (20mg) and diclofenac (100mg) [see chapter 6, fig. 6.1].

4) In the presence of an active peptic ulcer all NSAIDs are contraindicated and even suppositories or enteric-coated preparations may delay healing, but the NSAIDs least likely to cause dyspepsia and erosive bleeding are probably diflunisal, sulindac, fenbufen and ibuprofen, Two of these, sulindac and fenbufen, are 'prodrugs' not exerting their antiprostaglandin effect until metabolized in the liver.

5) With a wide range of NSAIDs at their disposal most practitioners will settle for 4 or 5 which have been available for some years and with which they have greater personal experience. It is only after wide general usage that rare side effects become apparent and the relative frequency of more common ones are evaluated. In Great Britain, the most frequently prescribed are indomethacin, naproxen, piroxicam and ibuprofen, all of which have been widely used for more than 3 years; aspirin in its different forms would certainly appear high on this list but as it is obtainable over the counter as well as on prescription exact figures are not available.

6) In the treatment of gout, the NSAIDs are, in my opinion and those of most of my colleagues, the drugs of choice. They are more effective than colchicine with fewer side effects and do not have the endocrine effects of the corticosteroids, corticotropin or tetracosactrin. In my experience, these drugs, while effective in resistant cases, on withdrawal are not infrequently followed by a return of symptoms. Such an effect is unusual with NSAIDs if they are gradually withdrawn at the end of an attack. The NSAIDs should be started early in the attack and administered at full dosage over the first 24 hours. Although colchicine is widely used to cover the institution of long term agents such as probenecid, sulfinpyrazone or allopurinol to prevent the occurrence of acute attacks at this time, the NSAIDs, at daily dosages lower than those used to treat gout, may be used in a similar fashion.

While any of the more effective non-salicylate NSAIDs may be used with effect in an acute attack those approved in Great Britain for the treatment of acute gout have been indomethacin, naproxen, sulindac, azapropazone, diclofenac, piroxicam and phenylbutazone (now withdrawn), but several studies have shown others also to be effective.

7) In ankylosing spondylitis, as in gout, the NSAIDs soon became the drugs of first choice as they relieved the painful stiffness of this condition better than simple analgesics and did not have the endocrine effects of the corticosteroids. Under cover of an effective well-tolerated NSAID the spondylitic patient is able to move more freely with less pain by day and has better nights and less morning spinal stiffness, though the evening dose may have to be increased if evening and early morning symptoms are severe. Phenylbutazone, when introduced in 1952, almost overnight became the drug of first choice in this condition (for which it is still approved) and in gout.

8) In rheumatoid arthritis, in addition to physical measures and general education of the patients in their own treatment, the NSAIDs are first-line therapy and the decision which one of them to use will depend on effectiveness and tolerance. As stated above, indomethacin, naproxen, piroxicam and ibuprofen, respectively, are the most prescribed NSAIDs in Great Britain, but the field is, happily, a large one. Aspirin in its different forms also comes high on this list.

9) In osteoarthritis the NSAIDs often given more symptomatic relief than simple analgesics, particularly when acutely painful inflammatory episodes occur. If a chosen NSAID does not produce a definite lessening of symptoms within 3 weeks, it should be changed to another, but if 2 or 3 NSAIDs in succession fail to relieve symptoms, they should be discontinued. In many cases, NSAIDs make life reasonable for the patient when hips or knees are severely affected and often can be used for several years before joint replacements are performed.

10) In seronegative inflammatory arthropathies other than ankylosing spondylitis the NSAIDs play a useful part; Reiter's syndrome, psoriatic arthritis and colitic arthritis, for instance, respond symptomatically in many, if not most, cases.

11) Back pains and soft tissue lesions such as the painful stiff shoulder may benefit from NSAID administration, but rather less than other conditions.

Physiotherapy, rest, injections of corticosteroids, analgesics and other measures are, on the whole, more helpful although the NSAIDs still have a part to play.

References

Altman, R.D. and Hochberg, M.C.: Degenerative joint disease. Clinics in Rheumatic Diseases 9: 681-693 (1983).

Ansell, B.A.: Juvenile chronic arthritis; in Hart (Ed.) Drug Treatment of the Rheumatic Diseases, 2nd ed., p.185 (ADIS Press, Auckland 1982).

Australasian Multicentre Trial Group: The simultaneous assessments of 4 non-steroidal anti-inflammatory drugs in rheumatoid arthritis using a simple and rapid trial design. Journal of Rheumatology 7: 857-864 (1980).

Baber, N.; Halliday, L.; van den Heuvel, W.J.A.; Walker, R.; Sibeon, R.; Keenan, J.; Littler, T. and Orme, M.L.: Indomethacin in rheumatoid arthritis: Clinical effects, pharmacokinetics and platelet studies in responders and non-responders. Annals of the Rheumatic Diseases 38: 128-136 (1979).

Bombadier, C.; Tugwell, P.; Sinclair, A.; Dok, C.; Anderson, G. and Buchanan, W.W.: Preference for endpoint measures in clinical trials: Results of structional workshops. Journal of Rheumatology 9: 798-801 (1982).

British National Formulary, No.7, pp.6 and 14 British Medical Association and Pharmaceutical Society of GB (1984).

Caruso, I. and Bianchi Porro, G.: Gastroscopic evaluation of anti-inflammatory agents. British Medical Journal 280: 75-78 (1980a) and 646 (1980b).

D'Arcy, P.F.: Fatal anaphylactic reactions with zomepirac. Pharmacy International 4: 99-100 (1983).

Doyle, D.V.; Dieppe, P.A.; Scott, J. and Huskisson, E.C.: An articular index for the assessment of osteoarthritis. Annals of the Rheumatic Diseases 40: 75-78 (1981).

European Rheumatism Council: Gold therapy in rheumatoid arthritis. Annals of Rheumatic Diseases 19: 95-119 (1960).

Fowler, R.W. and Arnold, K.G.: Non-steroidal analgesic and anti-inflammatory agents. British Medical Journal 287: 835 (1983).

Gall, E.P.; Caperton, E.M.; McComb, J.E.; Nessmer, R.; Multz, C.V.; O'Hanlan, M. and Wilkens, R.I.: Clinical comparison of ibuprofen, fenoprofen, calcium, naproxen and tolmetin sodium in rheumatoid arthritis. Journal of Rheumatology 9: 402-407 (1982).

Hart, F.D.: Rheumatic disorders; in Avery (Ed.) Drug Treatment, 2nd ed., pp. 846-888 (ADIS Press, Sydney 1980).

Hart, F.D. (Ed.): Drug Treatment of the Rheumatic Diseases, 2nd ed., p.2 (ADIS Press, Auckland 1982).

Hart, F.D. and Huskisson, E.C.: Non-steroidal anti-inflammatory drugs: Current status and rational therapeutic efficacy. Drugs 27: 232-255 (1984)

Heller, C.A.; Stanley, P.; Lewis-Jones, B. and Heller, R.F.: Value of x-ray examinations of the cervical spine. British Medical Journal 287: 1276-1278 (1983).

Huskisson, E.C.; Woolf, D.L.; Balme, H.W.; Scott, J. and Franklyn, S.: Four new anti-inflammatory drugs: Responses and variations. British Medical Journal 1: 1048-1050 (1976).

Lansbury, J.: Report of a 3 year study on the systemic and articular indexes in rheumatoid arthritis. Arthritis and Rheumatism 1: 505-522 (1958).

Luczynska, C. and Wilson, K.: The clinical significance of the effects of cigarette smoking on drug disposition. Methods and Findings in Experimental and Clinical Pharmacology 5: 479 (1983).

Mallya, R.K. and Mace, B.E.W.: The assessment of disease activity in rheumatoid arthritis using a multivariate analysis. Rheumatology and Rehabilitation 20: 14-17 (1981).

Mason, R.M.; Barnardo, D.E.; Fox, W.R. and Weatherall, M.: Assessment of drugs in out-patients with rheumatoid arthritis. Annals of the Rheumatic Diseases 26: 373-388 (1967).

Nuki, G.: Non-steroidal analgesic and anti-inflammatory agents. British Medical Journal 287: 39-43 (1983).

Oldham, R.: Gastroscopic evaluation of anti-inflammatory agents. British Medical Journal 280: 162 (1980).

Orme, M.; Baber, N.; Keenan, J.; Halliday, L.; Sibeon, R. and Littler, T.: Pharmacokinetics and biochemical effects in responders non-responders to non-steroidal anti-inflammatory drugs. Scandinavian Journal of Rheumatology (Suppl. 39): 19-27 (1981).

Paulus, H.E.: Rheumatoid arthritis – anti-inflammatory drugs. Clinics in Rheumatic Diseases 9: 571-580 (1983).

Rake, G.W. and Jacobs, R.L.: Anaphylactoid reactions to tolmetin and zomepirac. Annals of Allergy 50: 323-325 (1983).

Reynolds, P.M.G. and Whorwell, P.J.: A single blind cross over comparison of fenoprofen, ibuprofen and naproxen in rheumatoid arthritis. Current Medical Research and Opinion 2: 461-463 (1974).
Ritchie, D.M.; Boyle, J.A.; McInnes, J.M.; Jasani, M.K.; Dalakos, T.G.; Grieveson, P. and Buchanan, W.W.: Clinical studies with an articular index for the assessment of joint tenderness in patients with rheumatoid arthritis. Quarterly Journal of Medicine 37: 393-406 (1968).
Short, C.C. and Bauer, W.: The course of rheumatoid arthritis in new patients receiving simple medical and orthopedic measures. New England Journal of Medicine 238: 142 (1948).
Silvoso, G.R.; Ivey, K.J.; Butt, J.H.; Lockard, O.O.; Holt, S.O.; Sisk, C.; Baskin, W.V.; Mackercher, P.A. and Hewett, J.: Incidence of gastric lesions in patients with rheumatic disease on chronic aspirin therapy. Annals of Internal Medicine 91: 517-520 (1979).
Smyth, C.J. and Percy, J.S.: Comparison of indomethacin and phenylbutazone in acute gout. Annals of the Rheumatic Diseases 32: 351-354 (1973).
Vallance, J.: Statistical procedures in clinical trials. Master's Thesis, New South Wales Institute of Technology (1982).
Verbeeck, R.K.; Blackburn, J.L. and Loewen, G.R.: Clinical pharmacokinetics of non-steroidal anti-inflammatory drugs. Clinical Pharmacokinetics 8: 297-331 (1983).
Whitehouse, G.H. and Hart, F.D.: Indomethacin suppositories for arthritis. British Medical Journal 2: 427 (1965).
Yeung Laiwah, A.C. and Mactier, R.A.: Antagonistic effect of non-steroidal anti-inflammatory drugs on frusemide-induced diuresis in cardiac failure. British Medical Journal 283: 714 (1981).

Round Table Discussion

Panel

Dr Hedley Berry
King's College Hospital, London, England

Professor J.J. de Blécourt
University of Groningen Hospital, Groningen, The Netherlands

Dr P.D. Fowler
Staffordshire Rheumatology Centre, Stoke-on-Trent, Staffordshire, England

Dr F. Dudley Hart
Chelsea Hospital for Women, Westminster Hospital, London, England

Professor J.R. Klinenberg
UCLA Medical School, Los Angeles, California, USA

Dr Odd Kogstad
Aust-Agder Central Hospital, Arendal, Norway

Dr J.M.H. Moll
Sheffield Centre for the Investigation and Treatment of Rheumatic Diseases, Sheffield, England

Dr A.G. Mowat
Nuffield Orthopaedic Centre, Oxford, England

Professor A. Simkin
School of Medicine, University of Washington, Seattle, Washington, USA

Professor J. Villiaumey
Hôpital Henri Mondor, Créteil, France

Professor F. Wollheim
University Hospital of Lund, Lund, Sweden

NSAID Clinical Trials

Professor Klinenberg: *Dr Mowat, I believe you would agree that to provide tolerability data and to confirm long term efficacy, a long term study in a large population, treated with a single dose (or a narrow dose range) is essential. Very few such trials are published – what are the practical problems associated with them?*

Long Term Studies

Dr Mowat: The main difficulties are:

1) Recruitment of sufficient numbers.

2) Avoidance of too many assessment centers.

3) Measurement of efficacy. This is more difficult than recording side effects – general practice trials are almost useless as they concentrate on side effects.

4) Patient and assessor stamina!

Dr Kogstad: I believe there are additional problems of natural variations in disease activity which influence dosage and patient compliance. Patients are liable to take lower doses or stop medication altogether during periods of remission and may increase their dosage when the disease worsens. The tolerability of a drug also influences compliance and severe side effects will result in 'drop-outs' from the trial.

Dr Fowler: In my experience so-called large-scale studies, even in the largest instances, involve only thousands of patients treated for a few weeks. These will rarely show up the rare, very serious reactions, such as aplastic anemia, occurring in 1/50,000 'patient-months' of treatment; they are liable to misinterpretation.

Long term studies with narrow fixed dose ranges are totally impracticable in rheumatic disease, especially rheumatoid arthritis. In all but the mildest disease, our own and other studies have shown that fixed dose therapy is inadequate.

Postmarketing Surveillance

The efficacy of NSAIDs can be established in short term studies. There is no evidence that this diminishes with long term use, though the dose may vary. The only practical satisfactory way of monitoring long term safety is 'pharmacoepidemiology', the most cost-effective being the prescription-event monitoring scheme developed at Southampton by Professor W.H.W. Inman[1].

Dr Berry: I think it is important not to beat about the bush here. This sort of trial really does not confirm efficacy because, by its very nature, it is going to be 'open'. Open trials do not really reveal efficacy but may be useful in identifying toxicity, especially if the patient population is large enough.

---

1 Inman, W.H.W.: Postmarketing surveillance of adverse drug reactions in general practice. II: Prescription-event monitoring at the University of Southampton. British Medical Journal 282: 1216-1217 (1981).

Professor Wollheim: Another difficulty which arises in some countries is that postmarketing surveys are discouraged by some drug monitoring authorities, for example the piroxicam study in Sweden in 1983.

Professor Klinenberg: It is often difficult to determine what the best 'single dosage' (or narrow dose range) might be, since higher doses tend to provide greater efficacy but are less tolerable and the smaller doses, which are more tolerable, are frequently not as efficacious. Thus, the final decision on a dose comes after only many studies have already been completed and usually represents a compromise.

Furthermore, if one really does want to prove efficacy it is necessary to do a study over a very long period. Shorter studies may prove some efficacy with regard to symptomatic relief but if one wants to determine whether a drug influences the natural history of a disease, then the study must be over a 3- to 5-year period.

Professor de Blécourt: In my view, the major practical impediment to such long term studies is the impossibility of ensuring patients' compliance with the chosen regimen.

Can NSAIDs Be Disease-modifying?

Professor Simkin: *One or two of the newer NSAIDs are said to have shown some sign of a disease-modifying effect. How good is this evidence, and is it by chance that these drugs have been withdrawn from general use?*

Dr Fowler: Our own studies in Stoke have convincingly demonstrated a disease-modifying effect of benoxaprofen[1] and fenclofenac[2], as shown by a rapid decrease of ESR and C-reactive protein levels.

No, it is not by chance that these drugs have been withdrawn. Their adverse effects profile was compared with that of simple NSAIDs; it should have been compared with that of gold or penicillamine. Furthermore, they had been extensively prescribed in situations when they were not really indicated, for example the use of benoxaprofen in geriatric osteoarthritis.

Dr Berry: In our studies, originally on alclofenac and then on fenclofenac, we were able to show that these two agents were capable of causing a statistically significant reduction in ESR, a rise in hemoglobin, and a decrease in C-reactive protein and other acute phase reactants. The results were comparable with those of penicillamine but we had few patients, there were few withdrawals and the trials, although designed as pilot studies, were open to criticism. However, our work with alclofenac was subsequently confirmed by the London Hospital study which was never published, and our work with fenclofenac was confirmed by two other studies, one in the United Kingdom and one in Denmark.

In a further study, we compared benoxaprofen and chloroquine in rheu-

---

1 Shadforth, M.F.; Crook, P.R. and Fowler, P.D.: The effect of benoxaprofen on the clinical and serological effects of R.A. Comparison with chloroquine and dapsone. Proceedings of the VIIth Pan-American Congress of Rheumatology, Washington, p.S 121 (1982).

2 Unpublished data.

matoid arthritis for two years, and found them to be equally potent. On withdrawal from benoxaprofen, patients subsequently had flares in their arthritis which necessitated gold or penicillamine treatment. Thus, we feel that there is good evidence that all three drugs had some disease-modifying potential.

It is unfortunate that all have been withdrawn. I suspect it is by chance that this happened, although there were consistent side effects such as a higher incidence of skin rashes than is found with other NSAIDs. However, in all honesty, I do not believe that this is other than by chance.

Professor Wollheim: One is tempted to believe at this stage that the price of a 'disease-modifying effect' among NSAIDs is unacceptable toxicity. However, in my view, the documented evidence for this disease-modifying effect of benoxaprofen was not convincing. Regarding fenclofenac's potential, there are conflicting reports in the literature.

Professor Villiaumey: To say that any NSAID has a disease-modifying effect seems to me to be a very risky statement. It is well known how difficult it is to be able to state that any specific drug can change the course of a rheumatic disease. The number of such agents is very limited. Studies, stringent in methodology, and of long duration, are necessary before it is possible to make any such claim for a new NSAID.

Dr Dudley Hart: I doubt whether there is any connection between the fact that both alclofenac and fenclofenac were claimed to affect the disease process and both were withdrawn largely because of skin rashes. It is interesting to note that both penicillamine and gold also cause rashes but these are probably different. Alclofenac and fenclofenac were withdrawn because it seemed that their therapeutic advantages did not outweigh the toxic disadvantages – mainly skin reactions. The quick answer here is yes, it does seem to have been a chance happening.

Professor Klinenberg: I agree. Convincing evidence for a disease-modifying effect is lacking.

Therapeutic Dilemmas in Rheumatoid Arthritis

Dr Mowat: *What are the implications for the treatment of the newly diagnosed patient in view of the high rate of spontaneous remission of rheumatoid arthritis during the first year?*

Spontaneous Remission

Dr Dudley Hart: There are two approaches here. The first is to treat symptomatically using general measures and NSAIDs in the standard manner. The alternative approach is to increase the possibility of remission by giving SAARDs, such as gold salts or penicillamine, early in treatment. Most physicians favor the former approach. There is no real evidence that the latter method works and to prove or disprove the efficacy of this approach would require the almost impossible – a large, well coordinated multicenter trial with large numbers of patients.

Dr Moll: I agree with:

1) Conservatism in introducing potentially toxic agents.

2) Preference in the first instance for more 'benign' medication such as NSAIDs. However, each patient has to be considered individually, and clinical grounds will dictate therapeutic judgement, not statistics.

Professor Klinenberg: If one begins so-called remittive therapy during the period when high rates of spontaneous remission may occur, then when the patient does remit it is impossible to know the cause. After the first year I believe it is a different matter.

Professor de Blécourt: I agree. I adopt a conservative approach for the first 6 months.

Professor Villiaumey: Rheumatoid arthritis is evolutive; the first years are very often a succession of periods of worsening symptoms and spontaneous remissions. This argues for prudence in assessing the results of any treatment given during this first period. If an apparent improvement is to be attributed to treatment the benefit must have been achieved quickly and in a very much shorter time frame than would be possible as a result of spontaneous variations in the disease. However, interpretation can be based only on one's own practical experience. This is equally true of drug treatment given during phases of remission or worsening symptoms.

Peptic Ulcer

Dr Dudley Hart: *I often feel that gastric surgery may be the safest way of treating a patient with active rheumatoid arthritis who also has an active peptic ulcer, but what do others consider the best approach? Are H_2-receptor antagonists, such as cimetidine or ranitidine, given with NSAIDs an acceptable alternative in patients who might otherwise be denied NSAIDs?*

Dr Fowler: In mild cases avoid all NSAIDs and use simple analgesics alone – e.g. acetaminophen (paracetamol). If this is insufficient NSAIDs may be administered rectally, the best being naproxen or diclofenac suppositories.

In addition, I would use cimetidine 800mg at night for patients with active or recently active peptic ulceration. If additional suppressive medication is needed I would use gold because it is administered by the intramuscular route and itself rarely causes gastric upset.

Dr Mowat: I would use H_2-blockers. There is no evidence that NSAIDs and H_2-blockers interfere with each other's action and ulcers heal with concurrent usage[1].

Professor Wollheim: My approach would be to hospitalize the patient and then use H_2-receptor blockers, PGE_2 if available and acetaminophen. If NSAIDs are necessary I would use the lowest possible dose of rectal indomethacin. Parenteral administration may also be useful in these circumstances but this needs confirmation.

---

1 Crocker, J.R.; Cotton, P.B.; Boyle, A.C. and Kinsella, P.: Cimetidine for peptic ulceration in patients with arthritis. Annals of the Rheumatic Diseases 39: 275-278 (1980).

Professor Villiaumey: Practical experience seems to show that treatment of an active peptic ulcer by H_2-receptor antagonists allows concurrent treatment with NSAIDs and inhibits the harmful effects of NSAIDs on the gastrointestinal tract. The H_2-antagonists must, however, be given in sufficient doses and for as long as the anti-inflammatories are given.

Dr Moll: I think that the practice of administering combined NSAIDs and H_2-blockade should be avoided if possible and temporary discontinuation of NSAID therapy is preferable. If this is not possible, I would seek preparations designed to minimize gastrointestinal irritation, e.g. prodrugs, coated preparations or suppositories. Whatever decision is taken, such patients will need careful monitoring.

Professor Klinenberg: My approach would be to use parenteral gold which has very little, if any, gastrointestinal toxicity. However, if the patient is either allergic to or unresponsive to gold, then there are serious problems. Hydroxychloroquine or penicillamine might be tolerated as a slow-acting remittive agent but for the immediate symptomatic management of the patient one must either use small doses of corticosteroids (which is probably the safest approach) or consider using an NSAID in association with an H_2-receptor antagonist.

In patients with a history of ulcer disease, co-prescription of H_2-receptor antagonists seems to be acceptable for those who might otherwise be denied NSAIDs. There is less certainty that this combination will be effective in those who have active ulcer disease.

Professor de Blécourt: I too would give parenteral gold together with an antiulcer regimen.

Professor Simkin: Endoscopic surveys suggest that all of us sometimes use NSAIDs in patients with erosive gastritis and most of these people clearly do well. Nevertheless, demonstration of a gastric ulcer would contraindicate the use of any oral NSAID other than enteric-coated preparations. I am not aware, however, of scientific evidence or of a convincing rationale that would prohibit NSAID use in patients with duodenal ulcer disease. Such lesions are probably coincidental with NSAID therapy, which need not necessarily be altered in the presence of an effective antiulcer regimen.

Design or Trial and Error?

Professor Klinenberg: *There seems to be little evidence of how the chemical structure of an NSAID influences its toxicity or efficacy. It may be that the chemical structure influences things like half-life and plasma concentration and, in fact, these may then have an effect on the safety or efficacy of the agent, but to date there seem to be no good clinical correlates between the two, do there?*

Structure-activity Relationships

Dr Dudley Hart: Certainly the stereochemistry of NSAIDs is important in determining their actions and disposition. It is known that the arylpropionic acid derivatives (see p.11) possess a chiralcenter; the activity of these drugs resides in the sinister (S) configuration and the inactive rectus (R) enantiomer appears to undergo metabolic inversion to the S-form *in vivo.* Most of these drugs, with the exception of naproxen, are used as racemic mixtures; is it possible that intersubject variation in the clinical efficacy, tolerability and plasma concentrations may be due, in part, to differences in the rate and extent of this stereochemical conversion?

Professor Wollheim: This is entirely possible and, in any case, administration of pure S-isomers would be advantageous in lowering total body load of the drug. Excretion may involve active renal transport and thus be stereospecific. The problem will be actively investigated, no doubt, in the near future.

Analgesic: Anti-inflammatory Ratio

Professor Klinenberg: *Dr Dudley Hart, could one possible explanation of variability in patients' response to NSAIDs lie in their differing ratios of analgesic : anti-inflammatory activity? Is testing of such a thesis a practical possibility?*

Dr Dudley Hart: In theory, it would probably be feasible to test such a hypothesis in a study comparing the response to an NSAID in active rheumatoid arthritis with that in the non-inflammatory phase of osteoarthritis.

Professor Klinenberg: There is probably some variability in patients' responses to NSAIDs based on the ratio of analgesic to anti-inflammatory activity. Diflunisal, for example, is generally thought to be a better agent in osteoarthritis, than it is in rheumatoid arthritis, and this could well be explained on the basis of its greater analgesic rather than anti-inflammatory properties. Some attempt to differentiate clinically between their analgesic and anti-inflammatory properties might be very useful if it were possible.

Professor Villiaumey: There is no particular difficulty in demonstrating the anti-inflammatory capacity of this or that drug. It is very difficult, if not impossible, however, to detect whether the anti-pain effect that is seen arises from the drug's anti-inflammatory activity itself or from a distinct analgesic capacity. In the pathology of rheumatism the difficulties are enhanced by the fact that most diseases causing painful disability are seen also to have an inflammatory element.

In practice, therefore, there is very little possibility of verifying the consequences of possible variations in the relationship between the analgesic and anti-inflammatory capacities of the various NSAIDs.

Tissue Penetration

Dr Moll: *What role does tissue penetration play? Is there a predictable relationship between the half-life and synovial fluid level or any evidence that the synovial fluid level somehow correlates with clinical anti-inflammatory activity?*

Professor Simkin: The relationship between plasma and synovial fluid kinetics of NSAIDs has been discussed (p.74) and presumably, similar patterns pertain in the interstitial fluids of other connective tissue. Thus, we can use the accessibility of synovial fluid to examine tissue penetration of individual drugs. Such data, however, are not helpful in predicting or comparing the anti-inflammatory effects of individual NSAIDs.

Dr Fowler: Obviously without adequate tissue concentrations there are no pharmacological effects. There is a predictable relationship with plasma half-life and synovial fluid concentration. My own work with fenbufen[1], diclofenac sodium[2], and 'Osmosin'[3] clearly confirms this. Drugs with a long plasma half-life have synovial fluid concentrations of about 60 to 70% of the plasma concentrations and follow the same pattern. In contrast, drugs with a short plasma half-life have prolonged synovial fluid concentrations, with higher levels in synovial fluid than plasma in the later phases. These studies adequately explain why diclofenac sodium, a short half-life drug, is effective when administered twice daily. It is not possible to correlate single time-point concentrations with clinical activity.

Prodrugs

Professor Klinenberg: *What evidence is there that the fact of being a prodrug* per se *confers clinical benefit? One has in mind NSAIDs such as sulindac or fenbufen.*

Professor Simkin: For a prodrug to have a significant therapeutic advantage, it must be preferentially converted to its active form at sites of inflammation. If the same conversion occurs at sites of potential toxicity, then there is no benefit from the prodrug formulation. This is the critical point that requires further study before such benefits can be considered established.

Professor Simkin: *Dr Mowat points out that the effect on prostaglandins is only one of a number of factors involved in the inflammatory response. How much is known about the action of NSAIDs on other inflammatory processes?*

Mechanisms of Action

Professor Villiaumey: It has been shown that NSAIDs perform their main anti-inflammatory action by inhibiting cyclo-oxygenase and reducing the for-

1 Fowler, P.D.; Hothersall, T.E. and Crook, P.R.: Fenbufen (Lederfen). Plasma and synovial fluid concentration of parent substance and metabolites. Proceedings of the XVth ILAAR Congress, Paris, June 1981. Revue du Rhumatisme et des Maladies Ostéo-Articulaires. Special issue: abstract no. 1019 (1981).

2 Fowler, P.D.; Shadforth, M.F.; Crook, P.R. and John, V.A.: Plasma and synovial fluid concentrations of diclofenac and metabolites during long-term treatment of RA. European Journal of Clinical Pharmacology 25: 389-394 (1983).

3 Fowler, P.D. and Dawes, P.T.: Osmosin: Its effect on plasma and synovial concentrations of indomethacin. European Journal of Clinical Pharmacology 27: 689-691 (1985).

mation of prostaglandins. But we know also that certain of them have the capacity to inhibit lipoxygenase and the formation of the non-cyclic derivatives which arise from the activity of that enzyme, and play a large part in the inflammatory process, namely hydroperoxides (HPETE), hydroxides (HETE) and leukotrienes.

Furthermore, NSAIDs oppose the liberation of lytic lysosomal enzymes by the stabilization of the membranes of the lysosomes; stimulate oxidizing phosphorylation by the mitochondria, thereby causing a loss of the tissue energetic reserves that are indispensable for the creation of inflammatory areas; and finally possess antihistamine, antikinin and antikallikrein capacities. All these phenomena have been demonstrated.

Dr Moll: As has been pointed out by others, the precise mode of action of NSAIDs is still controversial and, it has been suggested, biased according to specialty. To pharmacologists prostaglandins are important; to biochemists free oxygen radicals; to biologists lysosomal enzymes and macrophages; and to immunologists lymphocytes and their activation products. From a biochemical viewpoint, the kinin system is regarded by some as the second most likely site of action of NSAIDs, after the prostaglandin system.

Ulcerogenicity

Dr Berry: *The animal data of Rainsford have been quoted as suggesting that the NSAIDs most likely to induce ulcer formation are those most likely to decrease gastric mucosal levels of prostaglandins. Is there any data from patients to suggest that this may happen clinically?*

Dr Mowat: No. I think that the prostaglandin story will fall flat. There are too many prostaglandins working for 'good' and 'bad' in the gastrointestinal tract. To concentrate on one or two will be a mistake. It is assuming and compounding the errors we have already made about NSAID actions on arachidonic acid metabolism.

Dr Fowler: Peptic ulceration is probably related more to dosage levels and duration of therapy, together with other drugs used, smoking, and genetic factors, than to the actual NSAID prescribed. Indomethacin – not the most effective antiprostaglandin drug in pharmacological terms – is probably the most frequent ulcer-inducer, maybe because it is used most widely. If I remember correctly, much of Rainsford's work has been done with animals stressed in most unusual situations – e.g. pigs stressed by suspension.

Dosage Considerations

Professor Simkin: *Under which circumstances might we expect that the presentation of an NSAID as a sustained-release tablet, suppository or plain tablet may make a difference to the therapeutic response?*

Dr Fowler: Years of clinical experience have convinced me that the slow-release indomethacin formulation is most effective for the relief of morning stiffness and pain. However, I cannot quote chapter and verse for references.

Dr Mowat: In the immediate treatment of pain the more rapid onset of action with a plain tablet is an advantage.

Dosage Form

Dr Dudley Hart: I can think of two situations in which sustained-release tablets or suppositories may be helpful. The first is when there is pain at night and early morning joint stiffness, as in active rheumatoid arthritis or ankylosing spondylitis. Sustained-release indomethacin or a suppository given at night can be of benefit. The other group of patients who may benefit from rectal administration are those who suffer dyspepsia with oral preparations or who have dysphagia, hiatus hernia or esophageal pouches or strictures. In addition to indomethacin suppositories, naproxen, diclofenac and ketoprofen are also available as suppositories in the United Kingdom.

Professor Klinenberg: In general, one might consider that plain tablets are usually most readily absorbed and that their effect is going to be the quickest. Sustained-release tablets per unit dose are released more slowly so that the onset is a little delayed but the effect is over a longer period of time. Suppositories might be more slowly absorbed under some circumstances. If, in fact, this is true for some acute inflammatory conditions, such as acute bursitis, tendinitis, or gout, one might wish to use an agent that is present in the highest possible doses as quickly as possible, and, therefore, might go the route of plain tablets or shorter-acting agents. For more chronic arthritides sustained-release tablets and suppositories might be of greater benefit – although the suppository is more an attempt to bypass the stomach as an alternative in patients who have direct gastrointestinal irritation from tablets or capsules.

Dr Berry: I think there are few situations where sustained-release tablet, suppositories or plain tablets make a difference to the therapeutic response as such. Part of the explanation for this is based on the misconception that all pharmacokinetics depend on blood levels. We consistently read about plasma levels and their relevance to clinical efficacy. The truth is that these are in all probability unreliable statements in that the therapeutic response seems much more related to synovial levels. There would appear to be reasonable evidence that you need a good peak and a long plateau in order to achieve adequate synovial levels, but the synovial levels may well last for a long time. Regimens which seem, on a pharmacological basis, to be curious medication may be perfectly acceptable. The trouble is that the ethics of repeated synovial aspiration make one anxious about studies aimed at working out dosage on this basis.

Chronobiology

Professor Villiaumey: *One hears a lot about so-called chronobiology and many patients with morning stiffness who are helped by an additional bedtime dose. What are the implications of this therapeutic approach if the NSAID chosen is one with a long half-life and, presumably, steady-state levels within the normal therapeutic range have been reached as a consequence of day-time symptom control?*

Dr Moll: If the drug achieves satisfactory anti-inflammatory control through its long half-life effects, one would expect chronobiological phenomena to be controlled accordingly – symptomatic 'spikes' being ultimately flattened as a steady-state is reached.

Professor Klinenberg: In general, patients with significant morning stiffness seem to do quite well on the long-acting agents which enable steady blood levels to be maintained over a 24-hour period. It is with the short-acting agents that the interval between the last dose at night and the next dose, possibly late in the morning, is too long. Patients who otherwise would go for up to 12 hours without medication seem to do better if they are given an additional dose of drug in the early morning hours or substitute a longer-acting agent for the last dose at bedtime.

Dr Kogstad: I think individual pharmacokinetic properties may influence this and that an additional bedtime dose may help morning stiffness in some non-responders even if steady-state levels have been supposedly reached.

Dr Dudley Hart: Just as a loading dose, particularly at night, appears to be more effective in early acute gout, the same applies with ankylosing spondylitis and rheumatoid arthritis if a short half-life drug is used as a 'lift' in the dose on retiring. When using an agent with a long half-life this should, in theory, be less necessary but in practice a nocturnal 'lift' is still beneficial.

Dr Berry: Again there seems to be this misconception that the plasma half-life is important. In my view, what is important is tissue half-life, and this idea that a slow-release preparation is going to give an advantage over a standard preparation is not based on clinical fact. The evidence for this is perhaps best illustrated with indomethacin in that an indomethacin suppository or capsule is at least as effective as a slow-release preparation for the relief of early morning stiffness.

Early Symptom Relief

Dr Dudley Hart: *Dr Moll, you have indicated that relief of symptoms is usually attained within 24 hours with indomethacin. What time lag can be expected with the other 'short half-life' drugs (i.e. 12 hours or less)?*

Dr Moll: In general, symptom relief (of pain and stiffness) is experienced after 24 hours, and often sooner, with other short half-life drugs. In some patients, benefit is experienced soon after the first or second dose of drugs given 3- to 4-times-daily. This response is doubtless governed by many factors, e.g. the type, severity, and duration of the inflammatory process, the dosage given, and the type of drug administered.

Professor Villiaumey: We do not consider there is any difference in speed of effect between indomethacin and the other short half-life anti-inflammatories, at any rate in clinical practice. However allowances must be made for this or that patient's sensitivity which may vary from one drug to the next. Moreover, chronopharmacology may also be involved in determining response.

Dr Mowat: There are several considerations here. Stable plasma levels and probably stable synovial levels are achieved after 4 to 5 doses, irrespective of a drug's half-life. Therefore a measurable response is a function partly of half-life but also of dose, but is not necessarily the *maximum* effect that will develop.

Plasma Concentrations

Professor Villiaumey: *Do plasma concentrations vary much among individuals receiving slow-release preparations of the short half-life drugs?*

Dr Kogstad: They vary to a considerable extent, because of pharmacokinetic differences, especially individual variations in absorption.

Dr Fowler: Our own work has shown that in single-dose studies there are wide variations among individuals, particularly during the absorption phase. With short half-life drugs in prolonged administration there are wide variations in the immediate post-dose period, but little variation thereafter for both active drug and metabolites.

Gout

Dr Berry: *In clinical situations such as acute gout, where a loading dose may be advisable, which factors are important in choosing an NSAID?*

Dr Fowler: Obviously any powerfully water-retaining drug (e.g. phenylbutazone) should be avoided if there is any cardiac failure. Rapid absorption and good gastric tolerance are the obvious requirements.

Dr Kogstad: I think there are several pharmacokinetic properties of an NSAID which are important when a loading dose is used, namely: half-life (absorption, distribution and elimination), bioavailability, protein binding, risk or drug interactions and danger of accumulation in renal diseases. Individual patient responses and the effect of age are also important.

Dr Dudley Hart: In general what we are looking for is a drug which will act quickly.

Dr Mowat: Although, traditionally, a loading dose is given in gout, I doubt whether it has the great effect on blood levels imagined. It may be largely wasted. Side effects may increase with dose, the important short term ones being on the central nervous system.

Professor Klinenberg: I believe it is probably best to use an agent with a shorter half-life. In the treatment of gout, where it is reasonable to get as high a blood concentration as possible initially, the loading dose should be with an agent which will not stay around for too long.

Professor Simkin: The choice, at present, is one of individual preference since neither the short- nor long-lived NSAIDs has clearly been shown to be superior.

Juvenile Arthritis

Professor Klinenberg: *In the treatment of juvenile arthritis might the longer half-life NSAIDs be of special value, Dr Moll?*

Dr Moll: The problems of parental supervision of antirheumatic drug therapy in juveniles, and compliance in juveniles old enough to take their own medication would seem to justify the use of longer half-life drugs to reduce the frequency of dosage – if, of course, they can be shown to be safe in juveniles.

Dr Kogstad: Long half-life NSAIDs may lead to better patient compliance especially in children. On the other hand, they may be more difficult to control in cases of complications and side effects.

Dr Dudley Hart: Ansell[1] reported favorably on the use of piroxicam, 10mg daily, in children weighing 30kg or less, but this was only over 2-week periods, although further studies are in progress. Ansell also approves the use of naproxen in children.

Once-daily Dosage

Professor Klinenberg: *Is once-daily dosing an unmixed blessing?*

Professor de Blécourt: There are no unmixed blessings in this world – nevertheless, I am in favor of once-daily dosing in rheumatology.

Dr Berry: No, it is not an unmixed blessing, it is a blessing for those patients in whom it is appropriate. There are others who find that once-daily dosage of an NSAID is inadequate and still need to take something extra last thing at night.

Dr Moll: Nor is it, in my view, as compliance may be imperfect in some patients, and a forgotten once-daily dose would deny them a whole day's medication; whereas missed doses in a multiple-daily-dose regimen would deny them only a fraction of their daily dose.

There may also be psychological advantages in taking a drug several times a day if patients perceive this as being more effective, or if it attracts opportunities for 'attention seeking'.

Professor Simkin: Not all rheumatic syndromes are characterized by unremitting, destructive, inflammatory lesions. For those which are not, there is no obvious need for round-the-clock NSAID coverage and periodic short-acting drugs may be entirely reasonable. This is often true, for instance, of osteoarthritis. Also, even when steady-state blood and tissue levels seem desirable, some patients with good self-discipline seem to derive placebo benefit from a regimen that includes more frequent than once-daily doses of medication.

Dr Mowat: There seems to be some suggestion that this may be an erroneous assumption. Indeed twice-daily dosage may equal greater compliance.

---

1 Ansell, B.M.: Juvenile chronic arthritis; in Dudley Hart (Ed.) Drug Treatment of the Rheumatic Diseases p.185 (ADIS Press, Auckland 1982).

Dr Fowler: I have strong views on this subject. There is no doubt that once-daily dosage greatly increases compliance for asymptomatic conditions such as hypertension, but patients with painful rheumatic diseases have an inbuilt 'compliance-alarm'! Furthermore, many of my patients have expressed anxiety when once-daily dosage has been proposed. 'What do I do if the pain comes back before the next dose is due?' I prefer traditional tid dosage for *rheumatic* complaints.

Dose in Relation to Meals

Professor Klinenberg: *Professor Simkin has advanced a logical case for giving NSAIDs before meals but many rheumatologists prescribe them with, or after meals. What do others think?*

Dr Mowat: I do not think there is *any* good reason for giving them with meals.

Professor Wollheim: I agree with Professor Simkin and, with the exception of aspirin, do not generally prescribe NSAIDs with meals.

Dr Moll: From purely clinical experience, taking NSAIDs *in relation to* meals is important.

Professor Villiaumey: Giving NSAIDs before meals, when the stomach area is not cluttered with food, certainly facilitates their absorption. It is then possible to give a smaller dose. But this is an advantage only in theory. The fact is that direct contact between NSAIDs and the gastric mucosa results in irritation which causes pain, a sensation of burning, and cramps and nausea, all of which considerably hamper the continuation of treatment. It is for this reason that numerous rheumatologists avoid prescribing NSAIDs on an empty stomach and prefer them to be taken during or after meals.

Dr Dudley Hart: There is obviously a great divergence of opinion on this subject and a multicenter trial to investigate the matter is probably indicated but I doubt whether there would be much enthusiasm to undertake it. Most textbook and product data sheets advise giving NSAIDs with, or immediately after, meals so they are less irritant though more slowly absorbed. This is current orthodoxy but Professor Simkin may well be right. A trial would have to include drug absorption (blood levels), clinical effects and gastroscopic studies. The latter alone would be helpful, and should be studied if it has not already been done: I will alert my fellow gastroscopists.

NSAID Side Effects

Dr Dudley Hart: *It has been suggested that the incidence of side effects from NSAIDs differs in rheumatoid arthritis as distinct from osteoarthritis and that patients with ankylosing spondylitis and gout have fewer side effects. Is this so and what are the likely reasons?*

Influence of Disease

Dr Fowler: There is no doubt about this, as my own published work[1] has clearly shown. There are two reasons. Patients with rheumatoid arthritis have prolonged therapy with many agents. In addition they have a systemic disease making 'organ' disease more susceptible.

Professor de Blécourt: My impression is that in the more active rheumatoid arthritis states side effects will be more common.

Dr Moll: One example of this phenomenon could be the apparent paucity of toxic effects in patients with acute gout, necessarily treated with maximal doses of NSAIDs. If this is a real phenomenon, perhaps the heightened inflammatory response in this form of arthritis 'soaks up' the drug more so than when there are lesser levels of inflammation. This would tend to reduce the amount of drug available for toxic effects.

Dr Berry: I am unaware of any such data. Certainly, it is not my clinical impression that this occurs.

Professor Villiaumey: No, I have never noticed such differences in my own experience either.

Professor Klinenberg: I, too, seriously doubt that for a given dose and duration, there is any difference in the incidence of side effects in patients with the various rheumatic diseases, all other things being equal, namely, the history of previous gastrointestinal diseases, etc. I think the *perception* that these drugs have fewer side effects in diseases such as osteoarthritis, ankylosing spondylitis and gout arises for the following reasons:

1) Gout is a very acute, self-limited disease and patients take NSAIDs for a very short period of time in any one attack. Thus, after 3 to 4 days of high-dose NSAID the dose is reduced to a small one or the drug is discontinued. Furthermore, the likelihood that the patient will respond to such therapy is very great. These patients also are otherwise healthy and do not have a multisystem disease.

2) Patients with ankylosing spondylitis also usually respond more quickly to NSAIDs than do patients with rheumatoid arthritis, and for that reason are much less likely to be exposed to ever-increasing dosage leading to ever-increasing toxicity.

3) Patients with osteoarthritis tend to have a very localized disease and are not systemically ill. Therefore, they might tolerate NSAIDs somewhat better.

Prescribing Habits

Professor Simkin: *Major toxicity is not common with NSAIDs. Is this because the newer drugs have a high therapeutic index or because clinicians are more conscious of the potential effects and how to avoid them, or a combination of both factors?*

1 Fowler, P.D. and Faragher, E.B.: Drug and non-drug factors influencing adverse reactions to pyrazoles. Journal of International Medical Research 5 (Suppl. 2): 108-120 (1977).

Dr Dudley Hart: Probably a combination of both. Major toxicity is still a problem as regards gastrointestinal hemorrhage or perforation but deaths due to other causes are rare as the newer NSAIDs are less toxic but still effective. Clinicians are more careful but the newer drugs are probably safer than the newer physicians!

Professor Klinenberg: Yes, I think both factors play a role: a relatively high therapeutic index with usual dosages which represent the lower end of the spectrum; and, since there are many drugs available, physicians tend to monitor their patients closely and to stop medication at the first sign of toxicity.

Dr Moll: I agree. Certainly in the days of widespread aspirin usage, clinicians became adept at seeking alternative preparations within the same generic group, and these were sometimes coupled with co-medication to minimize/abolish toxic effects; the latter being a more dubious practice in view of any 'painting-over-the-cracks' effect that may have delayed or prevented diagnosis of serious peptic disease.

Professor Villiaumey: There is no doubt that clinicians are better informed on the side effects of NSAIDs. They continue to mistrust them and to keep the same close watch over patients when they are under treatment with a new drug whatever they have been told about the supposed advantages it possesses. This attitude is all the more justified in that the very wide use of the new drugs after their launch on the market has, on several occasions, served to undermine the too optimistic opinions which resulted from early trials.

Dr Mowat: I feel that neither of these assumptions is valid. Much evidence points to bad prescribing – high doses, etc. – and yet few serious side effects. NSAIDs are essentially safe drugs.

Influence of Smoking

Professor Wollheim: *Dr Dudley Hart, are patients who smoke more liable to develop a gastric ulcer if they take NSAIDs?*

Dr Dudley Hart: I believe this to be so and unpublished work by Willoughby and Essigman has found some evidence of this. It has been shown that both smoking and NSAIDs are independently ulcerogenic so it seems likely that in combination they will have an additive effect.

Dr Fowler: It is worth pointing out that vasculitic ulcers may be another undesirable consequence of smoking in patients with rheumatoid arthritis. Clear evidence from Professor Bacon's unit in Birmingham has shown that vasculitic rheumatoid ulcers are in proportion to cigarette consumption. This was reported by Dr G. Struthers at a meeting of the Midland Rheumatological Society in 1983. My own subsequent clinical impression confirms this view.

Will Prostaglandins Help?

Dr Dudley Hart: *What about the new synthetic prostaglandins; are they likely to protect against NSAID-induced ulcer disease?*

Dr Mowat: No. To suggest that PGE_2 is the ideal 'good guy' is too simple.

Dr Kogstad: This is an interesting theoretical question; I do not think it will be a practical possibility, but this is a very active field of research.

Acceleration of Joint Changes

Dr Fowler: *Dr Moll, is there any evidence that NSAIDs accelerate the rate of degenerative change in joints?*

Dr Moll: Although some reports have suggested acceleration of degenerative changes in weight-bearing joints – especially the hip – this effect of NSAIDs continues to be hotly debated. For example, is the phenomenon due to a direct effect of the drug on the joint or is the increased mobility of patients so treated an indirect effect? Another school of thought doubts the significance of these changes, putting them down to chance.

Professor Klinenberg: There are animal studies, particularly in experimental osteoarthritis which suggest that using a joint during an acute inflammatory period accelerates the degenerative process, and, conversely, rest of the part helps speed healing. If one concluded that, in these animals, an effective NSAID would relieve symptoms thus enabling the joint to be used, then it surely would accelerate the rate of degenerative changes. I know of no human study which has shown that NSAIDs, in fact, do accelerate the rate of degenerative changes in any disease.

Dr Berry: I believe there is a certain amount of conflicting radiographic evidence that osteoarthritis of the hips may be accelerated by indomethacin. There is also mounting evidence from Professor Gabriel Panayi's unit at Guy's Hospital, London, that NSAIDs may worsen erosive rheumatoid disease, although this has been queried in some other centers.

Professor Villiaumey: On several occasions I have published observations on cases of coxofemoral arthrosis which rapidly deteriorated with indomethacin treatment. Various studies on laboratory animals have shown that this drug can influence the structure and metabolism of articular cartilage. However, in our studies in patients, the aggravation of anatomo-radiological changes in the hip seemed to be caused primarily by extra strain being put on lower-limb joints following pain relief and improved functional capabilities as a result of indomethacin treatment.

Thus, I believe that when any NSAID is used in the treatment of degenerative changes in the larger lower-limb joints: (a) only moderate physical activity should be undertaken; (b) dosage should be kept relatively low, allowing the development of minor pains to serve as an alarm mechanism for the patient; and (c) there should be occasional breaks in treatment.

Aspirin Hypersensitivity

Professor Simkin: *To what extent has the inappropriate use of NSAIDs in aspirin-hypersensitive patients contributed to the withdrawal of certain NSAIDs?*

Dr Kogstad: To a small extent in my opinion. Hypersensitivity to aspirin is relatively rare and hypersensitivity to NSAIDs, in general, is rarer. The concordance of sensitivity may not always be due to the same mechanism. NSAIDs that can be tolerated by aspirin-sensitive patients are also needed.

Professor Villiaumey: Although the prescribing information for a new NSAID invariably states that sensitivity to aspirin is a contraindication to its use, this may not be taken into consideration when the drug is generally prescribed. Such inappropriate prescribing may have been responsible for certain NSAIDs being withdrawn from the market.

Dr Dudley Hart: I feel that this certainly played a part in the withdrawal of zomepirac.

Newer NSAIDs

Professor Wollheim: *Is there any evidence that any of the new and investigational compounds such as fenbufen, carprofen or etodolac, have any clear advantage over more established agents such as naproxen and piroxicam in terms of their side effects?*

Dr Berry: The answer to this remains to be seen. Certainly fenbufen has no particular advantage and work with carprofen in the United Kingdom has been discontinued because of the high incidence of skin rash. As yet the situation with etodolac is unknown.

Professor de Blécourt: I know of no evidence so far which would point to these newer NSAIDs having any clear advantage.

Dr Kogstad: I would expect only marginal differences in the side effect profile of any of these; a drug has to be tested over years before any benefit can be shown conclusively.

Professor Villiaumey: Few controlled trials have compared the latest NSAIDs and older ones. Where this has been done, the dosage of the control drug was not correctly chosen, lying for instance at the lower limits of that customarily given for the disease under consideration. This meant that the results were more or less invalidated. In general, there is little evidence of one NSAID being actually better tolerated than another. The sensitivity of this or that patient seems to be the most important reason for variations in tolerance.

Renal Toxicity Less Likely with Sulindac?

Dr Moll: *It has been suggested that sulindac may be less nephrotoxic than other NSAIDs because of a more selective prostaglandin-inhibiting effect which leaves renal prostaglandins unaffected. Has this been proved clinically?*

Professor Simkin: No.

Dr Mowat: I agree. Any clinical effect is probably temporary[1].

1 Koopmans, P.P.; Thien, TH. and Gribnau, F.W.J.: Influence of non-steroidal anti-inflammatory drugs on diuretic treatment of mild to moderate essential hypertension. British Medical Journal 289: 1492-1494 (1984).

Dr Kogstad: To my knowledge there has only been one report of this, from Italy. It certainly needs confirmation.

Professor Klinenberg: There is significant evidence that sulindac's effect on renal prostaglandins differs from that of the other NSAIDs, and theoretically it should spare the kidneys. There is some anecdotal evidence that patients receiving sulindac have less renal toxicity and that patients who have had renal toxicity on other agents have done well when switched to sulindac. However, there has not yet been a major controlled study with sufficient patients to prove this point.

Dr Fowler: Nephrotoxicity is so rare that a significant clinical effect would be difficult to prove.

Media Publicity

Professor Klinenberg: *Dr Berry, a number of widely used NSAIDs have recently been withdrawn from the market in the United Kingdom. You seem to imply that the press had considerable influence on the decision to exclude these drugs. Should the public not be informed by the press of adverse effects to drugs commonly used to treat widespread diseases, providing that the medical profession and the pharmaceutical industry ensure that the information the press is given is kept in proper perspective?*

Dr Berry: I am sure the public should be informed of adverse effects to all commonly used drugs. On the other hand, there is a way of presenting the information which ensures that the public understands why the drugs are being prescribed and, as you say, the proper perspective kept. The big worry was that the information on benoxaprofen was not put over in the appropriate way, and the perspective was missing. This is why other compounds were withdrawn for insufficient reason. I think the media should be handled directly, but should be handled carefully and astutely by people who are trained to do so. The problem is that, on the whole, doctors in the United Kingdom have not been trained in media management and I feel that there are experts who are capable of either carrying out the role of the doctors in this area or even teaching doctors how they should go about it.

Dr Fowler: This is the subject for a book in itself! My colleagues at Stoke and I have published extensively on this subject[1]. However, there are misconceptions here. First, in our unit we are meticulous in advising patients about possible adverse reactions and both patients and their general practitioners are given information sheets when potentially toxic preparations, like gold or penicillamine, are prescribed.

Press reports of adverse drug effects are invariably exaggerated, for example, a report quoting 'over 400 deaths' with oxyphenbutazone failed to differentiate between oxyphenbutazone and phenylbutazone. Nor did it state that these had occurred over 25 years.

---

1 Dawes, P.T.; Fowler, P.D. and Hothersall, T.L.: An unhappy outlook for drug therapy. Lancet 2: 863 (1983).

Dr Mowat: Yes. I think the public is not involved enough in management. However it is a two-way trade. They should be told about side effects but, on the other hand, they need for their part to: (a) understand how a drug will benefit them; (b) take it properly; and (c) behave sensibly, e.g. with regard to diet, alcohol, smoking, etc., in relation to peptic ulceration.

Dr Moll: Yes, there is excessive publicity about adverse effects of drugs. Often this information is unduly alarmist and is aimed at a population of whom a large proportion will never be affected. And of course it is only right that individual patients actually taking drugs should be informed of more common toxic effects.

Professor Klinenberg: There is no doubt in my mind that the withdrawal of several agents in the United States has been the result of public pressure generated by articles appearing in the press. Many of these articles were based on only partial information, or were somewhat distorted. It is not an ideal way for people to be informed about adverse effects of commonly used drugs but it is the only one available. Surely we cannot suppress news or censor the press? The only solution is to try to keep the press as responsible as possible; to make sure that the pharmaceutical industry and physicians are willing to share with them enough information about drugs, their uses and toxicity so that patients can be given a much more balanced and reasonable accounting of both the benefits of and adverse reactions to the drugs we are currently using. Any attempt to suppress information is always viewed as a cover-up and will surely make the public more skeptical, making a bad situation even worse.

Subject Index